Introduction to Time-Limited Group Psychotherapy

Introduction to Time-Limited Group Psychotherapy

K. Roy MacKenzie, M.D., F.R.C.P.(C)

Professor of Psychiatry
Director of Resident Education
University of Texas at Houston
Houston, Texas

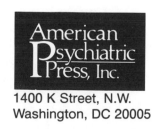

American Psychiatric Press, Inc.

1400 K Street, N.W.
Washington, DC 20005

Copyright © 1990 American Psychiatric Press, Inc.
ALL RIGHTS RESERVED
Manufactured in the United States of America
First Printing
93   92   91   90   4   3   2   1

The paper used in this publication meets the minimum requirements of American National Standard for Information Sciences—Permanence of Paper for Printed Library Materials, ANSI Z39.48-1984

Library of Congress Cataloging-in-Publication Data

MacKenzie, K. Roy, 1937–
    Introduction to time-limited group psychotherapy / K. Roy MacKenzie.
        p.   cm.
    Bibliography: p.
    Includes index.
    ISBN 0-88048-168-4
    1. Brief psychotherapy. 2. Group psychotherapy. I. Title.
    [DNLM: 1. Psychotherapy, Brief. 2. Psychotherapy, Group. WM 430 M156i]
RC480.55.M33   1990
616.89'152–dc20
DNLM/DLC
for Library of Congress   89-17508
                                                                             CIP

Contents

Section IV
Professional Practice

The past rides alongside the present and flails at it. In return, the present twists and reshapes the past for its own ends.

—Dennis Potter, BBC script writer and author of the "Singing Detective," as reported in the *New York Times* 07-10-88.

Preface

This book is designed as an introduction to group psychotherapy for the clinician who has had some experience with individual therapy. It is an introductory text but, because of the breadth of perspectives discussed, should be of interest to the more experienced group psychotherapist as well. Most of the material in the book concerns issues that are essential to the successful management of all types of therapeutic groups.

The understanding of group phenomena is approached from various points of view. The small group is considered as a complexly organized system. The influences of learning theory and social cognitive mechanisms are described, as well as the emergence of group norms. This group system is traced as it evolves through a developmental process in which a series of organizational tasks are addressed. The contribution of individual members is conceptualized in terms of social role functions. In addition to this basic small-group theory, an interpersonal psychodynamic perspective is added, which centers around focal issues that reflect past relationships of the individual that are reenacted in specific relationships within the group. The skillful management of these critical incidents permits the therapist to facilitate therapeutic learning. The integration of these various perspectives—systems theory, social psychology, learning theory, and interpersonal psychodynamic theory—creates a blend that is truly eclectic in nature.

The idea for this book originated in my experience in teaching introductory courses in group psychotherapy to psychiatric residents and other mental health professionals. I was particularly impressed by the lack of attention paid to basic group phenomena. I have tried to address this area with the material in Section I, "The Nature of Groupness," as well as in Section IV, where some clinically useful measures of group functioning are provided.

The clinical investigation of individual psychotherapy has developed considerably over the past decade. There is a growing consensus regarding important dimensions and successful therapeutic strategies. I have drawn from this literature when the material has seemed appropriate for understanding group therapy. This shift from a "clinical wisdom" approach to a focus on replicated findings has had a beneficial effect on psychotherapy teaching in general. One of my personal goals is to stimulate a similar process in the group therapy area. Considerable therapeutic mileage can be gained from the systematic application of a few well-defined concepts.

Although the ideas in this book are applicable to most group therapy situations, they are adapted particularly to circumstances in which the group will have a clearly defined life span. I have avoided using the term "brief" because it is quite variably interpreted. Time-limited groups have been described across a spectrum from highly structured groups of 8 sessions to groups running in seasonal terms from early fall to late spring, with perhaps up to 30 or 40 sessions. The important common issue is not the exact number of sessions but rather the intention that the experience will not continue indefinitely. The group developmental phenomena described later are seen most clearly in shorter-term closed groups, although the developmental perspective can be usefully adapted to other group formats as well.

Section I, "The Nature of Groupness," deals with basic ideas regarding the generic small group. It is written with the recognition that our society is filled with small groups that may have important healing or destructive influences on the participants. Formal therapy groups are subject to the same group factors. The ideas presented should allow the therapist to recognize these group phenomena and, in fact, to predict many of them. This can be a great reassurance as one begins the task of becoming a group therapist.

An effort has been made to identify specific behaviors or dimensions of interaction. These descriptions form observational guidelines for understanding and capitalizing on the use of established mechanisms by which groups can help people to change. By promoting and selectively reinforcing these activities, the leader can assist the group in reaching its full potential. Most therapists tend to think automatically in terms of individual issues. This may interfere with a full consideration of the power of a social system to mold and maintain behavior. The group perspective augments and expands the alternatives therapists have at their disposal for understanding behavior in a group. In particular, it may be helpful in distinguishing between individual pathology and normal reactions to stressful group events.

Section II, "The Early Group," applies the theories concerning time-limited group psychotherapy in a pragmatic clinical fashion. I have dwelt at some length on the early stages of a group, because in many time-limited group contexts the group's ending is inherent in its beginning. This section places great emphasis on the importance of assessment, composition decisions, and pretherapy preparation in ensuring that a sense of groupness will emerge quickly and bring with it a cohesive group atmosphere. The tasks of the first stage are concerned with ways to facilitate this process. The second stage of group development is described in terms of the differentiation process that underlies the appearance of conflict. Management guidelines as well as predictable problems are discussed.

Section III, "The Later Group," moves into more complex material. Section II dealt primarily with group-level issues, and the relationship of individual members to them. In Section III, the emphasis shifts into the management of individual issues using the emerging relationships among the group members as the vehicle for this work. The mechanisms of interpersonal learning are described in some detail. The activities and responsibilities of the group therapist as well as the basic style dimensions that have been found to effect group progress are described. The section ends with a chapter dealing with more personalized aspects of therapist functioning including a summary of situations that carry risk of producing negative effects. The material in this section has been influenced by the current interest in focused therapeutic techniques stemming from the individual psychotherapy literature. This material generally has not been applied in relation to group therapy, and I believe it is highly relevant.

In Section IV, a number of issues are addressed regarding the professional and service delivery context in which groups may be organized. This includes some information about group effectiveness, as well as practical topics of cotherapy, scheduling, and combining treatment methods. Guidelines for inpatient groups and long-term support groups are described. The implications for group psychotherapy of ethical issues, supervision practices, and training components are also reviewed. A method for keeping group records is described. The book ends with an overview of some simple clinical instruments that are available to measure change in individual patients as well as the more difficult task of measuring process events in groups. I call this approach "research with a small *r*." The intent of this material is to encourage the use of standardized measures to augment clinical judgment and to sharpen perceptions of discrete dimensions of group functioning.

The language used in the book is generally that of a medical setting. The ideas, of course, apply to participants of all therapy groups, who in some settings will be called *clients* or simply *members* rather than patients. I have also tried to avoid the use of professional jargon. This is in the service of the integrationist tradition that recommends the use of "plain English" rather than technical words associated with a particular theoretical orientation. The latter tend to be subject to simplistic assumptions, frank misinterpretation, and biased responses.

Rather than interrupt the flow of the text, I have deferred references to a special notes section where some introduction to the material is found. The selected references have been chosen with three criteria in mind: a publication of major historical interest in the development of group theory, a major review article, or a current publication reflecting emerging trends. My hope is that the introductory material in this volume will stimulate the reader to use this practical reading list as an introduction to the group psychotherapy literature.

To keep this a relatively brief general introductory text, a number of specialized applications for group psychotherapy have not been specifically addressed. The reader might wish to consult the publications of the American Group Psychotherapy Association Monograph series, which present more depth in selected areas: child group psychotherapy (Riester and Kraft 1986), adolescent group psychotherapy (Cramer-Azima and Richmond 1989), and group psychotherapies for the elderly (MacLennan et al. 1988). The *International Journal of Group Psychotherapy* regularly contains articles pertaining to specialized groups for particular patient populations.

Acknowledgments

During the preparation of this manuscript, I had occasion to reflect on my own development as a group psychotherapist. I would like to give recognition to some of the many people and experiences that have contributed to this. My interest was first whetted as a senior resident at the Mayo Clinic where I had the opportunity of participating in the early development of an intensive group-based day therapy program under the supervision of Dr. Loren Pilling. From those beginnings, I have had a long and rewarding association with the American Group Psychotherapy Association (AGPA). This organization serves as the major interest group for group therapists of many disciplines. The collegial relationships developed in that setting have been most rewarding. The heated discussions of the AGPA Research and General Systems Committees have been particularly thought provoking. Many years on the program committee gave me a unique opportunity to understand the diversity of approaches to group work. The opportunity of being a founding member of the Canadian Group Psychotherapy Association and serving as its president greatly extended my group psychotherapy world. Participation in local group psychotherapy societies in Calgary and Houston has given me an opportunity to understand the issues faced by group therapists in their daily work. Finally, I am appreciative of the feedback provided by numerous generations of trainees and have been gratified to see the interest generated for many of them in ongoing involvement in group psychotherapy.

I am particularly indebted to Fern Azima and Len Horowitz, who in different ways provided the opportunity for involvement in the organizational side of the AGPA. Maureen Coleman, who ably served for many years as coordinator of group psychotherapy in my program at Foothills Hospital, offered useful comments on this manuscript. My friend and colleague, John Livesley, also provided a helpful critique. Our association goes back many years to postsupervision sessions at "The Canny Man" in Edinburgh. My collaboration with Bob Dies in the first AGPA Monograph, "Advances in Group Psychotherapy," and subsequent work together on the editorial board of the *International Journal of Group Psychotherapy* have been greatly enjoyed and much appreciated. His careful review of early versions of this manuscript was particularly helpful.

The Nature of Groupness

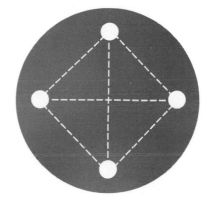

CHAPTER 1

Ideas About Groups

An understanding of therapy groups might begin with a consideration of the social behavior of the higher primates such as the chimpanzee and gorilla. Ethological studies demonstrate that biological mechanisms underlie the development of social interactional patterns. Two principal dimensions are described. The first is concerned with affiliation mechanisms that are associated with pair bonding, kinship societies, and the selection of sexual partners. The second dimension is concerned with the establishment of a dominance hierarchy and competition. These two axes provide a theoretical basis for understanding a great deal of primate social behavior.

The higher primates perform such complex tasks as the selection of leaders, negotiated coalitions, and scapegoating (redirected aggression). They also demonstrate social deception maneuvers and altruistic behavior. These require the ability to assess accurately the intentions of others, a necessary quality for the development of social relations. The addition of language and therefore symbolic associations produce more diversity in the meanings that humans attribute to social events. Nonetheless, the basic social enactment patterns appear to be closely related to those determined by genetic predispositions (1).

Throughout most of mankind's history, society has been organized on the basis of small to medium-sized groups. Natural leaders have generally been experts at managing group phenomena for purposes of political control, religious observance, social activity, or educational programs. The increasing role of group psychotherapy in contemporary Western society may in part be explained as a counterbalance to problems with the availability of indigenous social institutions. Social and demographic changes, such as increased mobility and the concentration of populations in large urban centers, have decreased the availability of established social organizations that have historically provided support and guidance.

The widespread use of groups as a clinical treatment modality stems from the wartime experiences of the 1940s. During this relatively brief period, group psychotherapy has become firmly entrenched as a component of psychiatric care. The formal conceptualization of group processes has developed only in the last century. The systematic use of groups in social and business contexts has also grown in significance during this same period. This chapter provides an introduction to the principal historical themes that underlie current group theory and practice (2).

Early Group Theories

The Danger of Group Emotion

Current theories about groups have evolved from ideas first developed early in this century that still influence our understanding of groups. These theories viewed the group as a potentially ungovernable force that had to be kept under control. At the turn of the century, LeBon wrote of the power of large groups to influence the individual member. This process of "mob contagion" under the influence of a charismatic leader was seen as a dangerous process. The civilized controls of the individual could be overcome by the "group mentality," resulting in a primitive impulse-ridden climate of intolerance, prejudice, and uninhibited behavior. It is interesting that, at about the same time, socialist theory spoke of the positive power of the masses and the value for the individual of being included in common goals. These divergent viewpoints reflect an increased appreciation of the power of the group to influence its members. The fear of emotional contagion is commonly found in patients approaching their first group session.

McDougall felt that the release of such "mob" processes could be controlled through group organization and task orientation. Even under these conditions, an intensification of emotional response would occur that required channeling into positive accomplishment. The role of the leader in structuring the group process was considered necessary to raise the collective mental life to a higher level. For both LeBon and McDougall, emotion was viewed as a dangerous and ungovernable force to be brought under control lest it result in the breakdown of moral responsibility.

Freud added further refinements to these ideas. He considered the essence of the group to stem from a common attachment to the leader, who represented the father figure—"A primary group of this kind is a number of individuals who have put one and the same object in the place of the ego ideal and have consequently identified themselves with one another in their ego. Thus, the common attachment to the leader provides a basis for group cohesion." This process permits a feeling of empathy and mutual identification among the members because of their common orientation. It also represents what today would be called a quality of universality, the experiencing of similar thoughts or reactions. At the same time, the idealization of the leader could diminish the individuality of each member and lead to domination by a powerful and charismatic figure.

Freud supported this theory by reference to his earlier hypothesis in "Totem and Taboo," in which he suggested a common genetic inheritance of the memory of the destruction of the father/chief by the younger men who then became a unified community of brothers. He viewed the tendency for members to become united in positive feelings toward the group leader as an illusion representing a reaction formation to the opposite state of affairs in the primal horde. In an idea never fully developed, Freud also pointed out the inverse relationship between neuroses and group membership. He suggested that an individual excluded from the group would be compelled to replace group relationships with neurotic formations. Freud's ideas have been elaborated by later writers, but he, himself, did not pursue their application (3).

Freud's views of the centrality of the leader in promoting a cohesive working group continue to be a source of controversy to this day. Leader-centered therapists conduct what amounts to individual psychotherapy in a group, with the setting providing an additional opportunity for members to learn from observing the experience of others. Group-centered therapists see the major curative factors in groups as stemming from member-to-member interactions, with the therapist's role being to develop and maintain a therapeutic group culture.

The Pragmatists

At an applied level, Joseph H. Pratt is sometimes cited as the first North American group therapist. He used an educative/inspirational model for improving the morale of patients with tuberculosis in Boston in the early years of the century. Trigant Burrow applied analytic ideas to groups in the 1920s. He was interested in the effects of social stress on physiologic tension and used group methods having much in common with later ideas about therapeutic communities. Over the next two decades, group experiences were reported by numerous practitioners, including E.W. Lazell, L. Cody March, Louis Wender, and Paul Schilder. They adapted group work in various ways to hospital settings, generally with the use of educational techniques combined with an awareness of group support factors. The efforts of these pioneers in group psychotherapy are important in retrospect, but, at the time, the use of group modalities was sporadic and outside of the mainstream of clinical work.

Analytic Ideas and Groups

In the postwar years, various ways of applying psychoanalytic principles to the group context were described. In America, S.R. Slavson was a proponent for the development of group therapy in the New York area, where he conducted children's groups in the prewar years. His organizational efforts resulted in the formation of the American Group Psychotherapy Association in 1942. In his application of ideas from individual psychoanalytic work to therapy groups, Slavson emphasized the importance of understanding emotional dimensions in the relationships of each member to the therapist and to other group members. The basis of his approach was the analysis of these group relationships through interpretations linking current neurotic behavior to early childhood experiences. Slavson recognized the importance of the diversity of relationships available in a group, but he placed priority on psychodynamic insight as the final common pathway to therapeutic change. His approach stressed the importance of the role of the leader in making accurate interpretations.

Slavson's position represented an important development for group theory. His writings reflect an appreciation of the group context and the diversity of relationships within it as a component of the change process. His insistence on interpretations directed at the individual led him away from conceptualizing the group as a system with its own potential for good or harm. He described therapeutic factors but considered them to be virtually identical to those found in individual psychotherapy. Thus Slavson made use of the group context but still saw the prime therapeutic influence as stemming from the leader.

Alexander Wolf and Emmanual Schwartz, contemporaries of Slavson, represented a somewhat different application of an analytic orientation. They paid greater attention to group factors that have a therapeutic effect. They saw more potential for learning from member-to-member interactions and cautioned the leader to hold back when such group work was being used effectively. Wolf promoted the idea of alternate sessions without the leader as a specific way of encouraging greater member initiative and responsibility. Fritz Redl described the importance of group emotional contagion and the role that different leadership styles of the "central person" may play in the nature of the group reaction (4).

The Social Psychology Research Tradition

Academic interest in small-group behavior began to develop in the 1930s and gathered momentum in the 1940s and 1950s. This research-oriented tradition existed in almost total isolation from clinical work. In fact, integration seemed to be specifically resisted by both sides. Analytically oriented practitioners felt that social perspectives were trivial in comparison with intrapsychic effects, and social psychologists preferred controlled settings to therapy groups for experimental manipulation. The work of the following three psychologists is representative of the social psychology tradition.

Kurt Lewin was interested in understanding the mechanisms at work in groups. His "field theory" is conceptually a precursor to general systems theory. The group is pictured as a field of competing needs or goal-directed behaviors. Each member must sacrifice some personal needs to meet the requirements of group membership. This process produces tensions between cohesive and disintegration tendencies. Lewin focused on the here-and-now group context as the best source of information regarding the motivations underlying overt behavior. Many of Lewin's ideas were incorporated into the programs of the National Training Laboratories in which the process of conflict resolution was carefully studied. This work led to broader use of experiential group techniques that were popularized through the "T-group" and "sensitivity group" activities of the 1960s and early 1970s.

Robert F. Bales pursued this theme concerning the tensions that might develop over conflicting needs in the group. He considered the resolution to lie in the development of a structural hierarchy that would at least bring predictability to the group process. This idea of conflict management provides a theoretical bridge between individual issues and group structure somewhat similar to McDougall's earlier theory of group task focus. Bales' system of Interaction Process Analysis has been used widely to study group phenomena. Each group action is placed into subcategories concerned either with task accomplishment or with tension management. Attempts to address the task tend to increase tension, necessitating reintegrative activity; but the work of pulling the group together distracts from task attention. Groups therefore cycle between task and socioemotional functions.

William C. Schutz incorporated some of these ideas into his own three-dimensional system for understanding human interaction needs for inclusion, control, and affection. The parallels between these interpersonal needs and the analytic ideas of oral, anal, and Oedipal phases of development can be seen as well as with Bion's "basic assumption" states of dependency, fight/flight, and pairing described in the next section. Schutz developed a measuring instrument called the FIRO (Fundamental Interpersonal Relations Orientations), which he applied to ideas of group composition and development (5).

Conceptualizing the Group

Before the war of 1939–1945, the formal use of group therapy was largely restricted to a handful of practitioners who applied the principles of individual psychoanalytic work to the group setting. Hospital-based programs made use of group activities and group educational approaches, but these contributed little to the development of group theory. The war created the need to treat large numbers of patients with stress-induced psychiatric disability. A group of British psychiatrists, who worked together in the Northfield Military Hospital, were responsible for capitalizing on these circumstances to develop new ideas about groups. These included ways of conceptualizing whole-group phenomena as well as thoughts about the hospital ward as a therapeutic community in itself.

The Group as a Whole

In terms of group psychotherapy, the principal figure from that group was Wilfred Bion. Bion stimulated a major theoretical shift in group understanding through a series of articles written between 1943 and 1952 that were eventually published as a book, *Experiences in Groups and Others Papers*, in 1961. This work is associated with the term *group-as-a-whole* school. Bion considered a group to be in either a "working" state or one of various "basic assumption" states. A working group has a clear idea of its tasks and is able to test rationally whether it is accomplishing them. The structure of the group is designed to facilitate cooperative task accomplishment, and various members become active in fulfilling helpful leadership tasks. This work group atmosphere may be interrupted by basic assumption states in which primitive drives and reactions prevent the group from maintaining its task-relevant activities (6).

The phrase "basic assumption" is used to describe a collective reaction of the members. It appears as if the members had arrived at some implicit understanding regarding the group's major problem at a given point in time. An analogy may be drawn between basic assumption phenomena in the group and resistance in individual therapy. Bion described three basic assumption states which he considered to be evidence that the group members are avoiding individual responsibility for therapeutic progress:

1. *Basic assumption dependency.*   The group acts as though it can only function effectively if a superior and wise person can be found who will lead it. Not surprisingly, the designated leader is often seen as the appropriate source of such leadership. Group members in this state behave as if they were helpless to direct their activities and instead address their problems from a position of passivity.
2. *Basic assumption fight/flight.*   Here the group clusters together as if threatened by a dangerous force. The language of the group centers around themes of threat and the need to defend itself or escape. There may be accusations about outside forces that are the locus of difficulty. Alternatively, individual members may be identified as the source of the group's problems. Such groups may experience rapid alterations between themes of fear and themes of revenge. The group may turn on the group leader for the failure to resolve issues and provide answers. A strong and absolute leader is sought.
3. *Basic assumption pairing.*   This is the most obtuse of Bion's descriptions. The group is preoccupied with issues concerning two of its members and acts as if a resolution of the problems presented by this pair would be of therapeutic value to the entire

group. This may have a voyeuristic quality with sexual overtones. As in the other two basic assumption states, the responsibility for direction is displaced from the individual member to another source.

Bion attempted to apply a psychoanalytic point of view in which the group is regarded as a quasi-individual with its own "group mentality." This mentality consists of disavowed dependent, hostile, or shameful parts that the individual members project into the collective space of the group. He considered each member to resonate to this central theme according to personal predisposition. There will be varying degrees of "valency" in the eagerness of members to respond to a given basic assumption state. The group will seek out and pressure those members most in harmony with the theme to serve as leaders. Thus, a member with a tendency to use projective defenses might be seen as a potential leader during basic assumption fight/ flight states. This group-as-a-whole approach shows the influence of McDougall's idea of group task organization as protection against destructive emotion, and the theories of Melanie Klein about primitive childhood defensive patterns.

The descriptions of the basic assumption states vividly portray common group experiences. They are useful as a signal that a group is moving away from productive work into a resistant or regressed position. They do not provide an adequate general theory of group functioning. The assumption that all members of the group are preoccupied with the same defensive posture seems unrealistic. Nonetheless, Bion's descriptions draw attention to the power of the group to influence the emotional responses of the members, particularly under adverse circumstances. This idea of the group as an amplifier of emotion is a useful core conceptualization. Bion's work continues the tradition of LeBon and McDougall in viewing emotion as a problematic phenomenon that is basically destructive in nature and requires control.

Bion worked for a time at the Tavistock Clinic in London, where he conducted groups using an unusual style of leadership. The leader would sit silent, not responding to questions, essentially unrevealing of personal responses, and making only infrequent group interpretations regarding evidence for resistive group behavior. A typical intervention might be, "The group is behaving as if it believed that I, the therapist, have a solution that I am keeping from the group (silence)." Not surprisingly, this style of leadership is effective in escalating the level of emotional arousal within the group. It often results in groups that become increasingly disorganized and angry. Follow-up studies suggest that therapy groups conducted using these leadership principles have the potential of harming some participants (7).

Bion's concepts continue to have an active life in group organizations. They are likely to be found in training groups using the label "Tavi" (Tavistock) or "group-as-a-whole" experiences. In North America, these are often sponsored by branches of the A.K. Rice Institute. Such group experiences can be of value for healthy participants who wish to learn more about group phenomena. They tend to deal predominantly with issues of control.

The Tavi leadership style is not congruent with the idea of a helping relationship. In therapy groups, positive cohesive dimensions must play a more central role. There is a danger that trainees who attend such group relations experiences may model the austere therapeutic style in clinical work. Tavi workshops provide an opportunity to learn about group dynamics, but should not be misconstrued as representing an effective style for therapy groups composed of dysfunctional patients.

The Idea of the Group Matrix

S.H. Foulkes was a British psychiatrist and the founding father of the British Group-Analytic Society. Foulkes applied analytic principles to groups in a different way from Bion. He stressed the importance of the group network and of understanding behavior in its social context. Where Bion understood "groupness" to stem from resistance, Foulkes emphasized the positive healing power of groups.

Foulkes used the term *group matrix* to describe the manner by which individuals develop their unique views of the group. The individual member participates in the creation of the current group at the same time attempting to reestablish the conditions of his or her own primary network as experienced in earlier life. Foulkes considered this to be the group equivalent of transference neurosis. By striving to understand each member's view of the others in the group, both members and leader, the therapist gains access to that individual's group matrix of personal interpretations. Conceptually, the "group" consists of the intersecting perceptions of the totality of its membership.

The analytic structural model of ego, id, and superego was superimposed onto the group. Through processes of splitting and displacement, the individual member's psychic life is re-created in the group, with some members coming to represent primitive wishes, others a parental controlling force, and so on. Thus, the group becomes a "hall of mirrors" reflecting internal states. This is a considerably broader application of analytic ideas than Freud's focus on reactions to the leader and Bion's concern with negatively valued aspects of self.

Foulkes emphasized the role of the therapist as a "conductor" who leads the group by following emerging material, who maintains an analytic attitude of nonjudgmental neutrality, and who avoids personal reactions or advice. He also spoke sensitively of the importance of an honest, genuine attitude on the part of the therapist, and of the primacy of experiential change mechanisms in terms very close to those used later to describe "therapeutic factors." His interest in the group matrix of each member led him to focus more on here-and-now group events than on genetic understanding of the family of origin. Foulkes' ideas provide a bridge between classical analytic ideas and current conceptualizations of the group as a therapeutic milieu (8).

Group Focal Conflict

Another major theoretical development that appeared in the postwar years was that of "group focal conflict." This idea grew from the writings of Thomas French in Chicago and Henry Ezriel in London. These authors conceptualized individual dynamics in terms of a nuclear conflict originating in early life experiences. French used the terms *disturbing motive* (a basic wish, need, or impulse) that produces a *reactive motive* (of fear or guilt), resulting in a state of tension demanding a *solution.* Ezriel described similar phenomena with the terms *avoided relationship* (the impulse), *calamitous relationship* (the fear), and *required relationship* (the defense, or solution). If the solution is adaptive, the competing motives are held in equilibrium and tension drops. If the solution is maladaptive, increased tension threatens to break through. This idea of a central conflictual theme continues to play a major role in the current literature on brief individual therapy under the title *interpersonal focus.* It is a theme that is taken up again in Chapter 6 (assessment) and in Chapter 10 (the advanced working group).

Ezriel conceived of the therapy group as a field of battle on which each participant tried to twist the others to meet personal needs regarding the satisfaction of conflictual themes. This process would result in the production of a "group focal conflict" theme that represented the common denominator of the dominant unconscious fantasies of all members.

Lieberman, Whitaker, and Whitman, originally at the University of Chicago, developed this concept of focal tension to the group setting. They looked for the emergence of common themes of concern from members of several groups. Once a theme was established, the group would try to find a solution to the conflictual problem in some way. Some solutions might focus almost entirely on the fears, without attempting to satisfy the associated shared wish. Other solutions may allow some expression or satisfaction of the wish. A "restrictive" solution deals only with the fear, which being contained, leads to a drop in tension. Such solutions restrict options and prevent resolution of the underlying conflictual material. In contrast, an "enabling" solution deals with the fear while allowing some expression of the wish. This reduces the tension level while at the same time permitting an exploration of associated impulses and feelings.

In the initial elaboration of this theory, it was assumed that all group members actively participated in the group focal conflict theme. This is analogous to Bion's idea of the valency, or strength, by which each member participates in a basic assumption state even though silent. In her later work, Whitaker implies that a particular theme may be relevant primarily only to a subset of group members (9).

These ideas of group focal conflict introduce into the group literature the concept of internal conflicts that are lived out through the group process. This is a broader position than that of Bion or Freud but perhaps less encompassing than Foulkes' notion of the group matrix. Although it is helpful to think of typical or central issues for each member of a group, it seems problematic to consider these as characteristic of the entire group membership. Because the number of core interpersonal themes is relatively limited, in any given group it would not be surprising to find some members reacting together around a common concern. Focal conflict theory is most appropriately applied to the individual. Individual members may then be compared or contrasted in terms of their focal themes. Ideas related to group development discussed in Chapter 4 suggest an alternative format for understanding content themes that arise in the group. The discussion of critical incidents in Chapter 10 suggests a different approach to managing group themes.

Current Theories

Therapeutic Properties of the Group

The idea that the group itself might provide a major component of the helping process began to emerge in the 1950s. This constituted a radical theoretical break from the analytic origins of group psychotherapy. In 1955, Corsini and Rosenberg reviewed the group literature, working on the assumption that beneath theoretical rationales there might be therapeutic mechanisms that were common to all group therapies. They looked for evidence of actual observable elements rather than theoretical constructs. This shift in perspective implied that the therapeutic power of groups did not lie solely within the activities of the leader role. Their pioneering work moved into the mainstream of group psychotherapy with the publication of the first edition of Yalom's group psychotherapy textbook in 1970, which placed major emphasis on what at that time were termed *curative factors*.

Yalom's book emerged in the context of major social change. In the professional literature this was reflected in many ways. Lewin's social psychological approaches were being widely implemented in sensitivity and encounter groups. Carl Rogers was working in "personal growth groups" using his client-centered concepts for providing a facilitating environment. Jerome Frank was simultaneously investigating the impact of "nonspecific factors" such as hope and acceptance in the helping relationship. Harry Stack Sullivan was developing his ideas about the interpersonal basis of psychological development. The ideas of this period conceptualized therapy, not as a search for pathology so much as a means of providing an opportunity for personal development. The distinction between therapy and a helpful experience became quite blurred. This positive orientation resonated with the social excitement and disruptions of a demographic swell in the numbers of young people (10).

Yalom's approach reflected this person-oriented tradition with roots in humanistic psychology. He placed greater emphasis on the importance of interactions among group members that promoted the operation of "therapeutic factors." The group was seen as a social microcosm with important therapeutic properties of its own. Genetic insight and therapist interpretations were downplayed as mechanisms of change in favor of interpersonal learning experiences in the current group interaction. This approach has had a profound effect on the general tenor of group therapy in North America that continues to the present. It exists today in a somewhat uneasy partnership with the psychoanalytic tradition that stresses the importance of leader-centered interpretations. Although the two approaches are not necessarily incompatible, there is enough difference in emphasis to cause a degree of polarization within the professional community. The interpersonal school describes the role of the therapist in creating and maintaining a therapeutic milieu within which therapeutic factors can be active. The psychoanalytic tradition views the therapist in the role of transference figure and interpreter of psychodynamic conflicts.

Action Techniques

A final important theme in the development of ideas about group psychotherapy has to do with methods that emphasize action over words. It is hardly surprising that such ideas have been readily incorporated into group work; after all, a group in one sense provides a built-in audience.

Jacob L. Moreno's psychodrama techniques originated in the 1930s. He opposed the analytic thinking of the day to promote the idea that man is a social being and therefore that the social system must be addressed to produce change. His techniques involved the acting out of distressful events or themes. Various group members might be chosen to represent important figures to be confronted, or as protagonists to speak on behalf of the patient. The important process was to re-create in the therapy room important transactions that could then be examined. In the process, personal or family secrets or secret assumptions might be laid bare for more objective consideration.

Gestalt techniques pioneered by Fritz Perls also used an action dimension. For example, the empty chair exercise consists of populating the chair with images of a significant other, or alternating occupancy of it to speak to both sides of an issue on which the patient is split. As with psychodrama, such methods translate internal states into action.

Taken by themselves, these action techniques tend to be used in the service of individual therapy in a group setting. Observing group members may benefit vicariously by seeing pertinent issues enacted, but the intent is clearly to deal with the individual in the spotlight. The incorporation of action methods into ongoing group interaction is common. Encouragement for a member to demonstrate issues, or speak to others as if they were family members can be smoothly integrated into more traditional group therapy formats. The action tradition is in keeping with the idea of using group process as the principal vehicle for learning (11).

The Integration of Ideas

For the last two decades, there has been an increasing emphasis on ways to integrate these various theoretical perspectives. The origins of this process arose earlier. For example, Hugh Mullan and Max Rosenbaum placed emphasis on greater therapist flexibility and decreased status level in order to promote more genuine "experiencing." Saul Scheidlinger worked creatively on integrating analytic theories with group dynamics. Henrietta Glatzer addressed the importance of the therapeutic alliance. These trends accelerated with the publication in 1964 of Helen Durkin's book *The Group in Depth*. This became one of the major texts in the field for many years. Durkin devoted a major section of her book to a review of the group dynamics literature and how it might be integrated into therapeutic work. Her ideas, 25 years later, still emerge as stimulating and provocative. Yalom's text in 1970 continued this integrative tradition, with a particular emphasis on using group research studies to justify clinical ideas. Currently, the integrative approach emphasizes the operation of common basic factors that cross theoretical orientations. Taken together, these appear to account for a much greater amount of therapeutic effect than specific techniques. These factors include the importance of the expectations brought by the patient, participation in an emotionally charged and confiding relationship, gaining an objective perspective on problems, having corrective experiences in the therapeutic setting, and applying these to real outside circumstances (12).

Recent trends in individual psychotherapy have been readily applied in group work as well. Therapists interested in self-psychology have been interested in the experiencing/accepting quality of the group environment. Those concerned with the perspective of object relations have emphasized strategies for selecting group, interpersonal, or intrapsychic levels of interventions. Psychodynamic psychotherapy has historically been applied in group settings. General Systems Theory offers a framework for integrating hierarchical levels of understanding as described in James Durkin's edited volume of 1981. These theoretical perspectives will be incorporated in later chapters (13).

Time-Limited Psychotherapy Groups

The idea of providing intensive therapy through time-limited group experiences is relatively new. Brief groups were initially thought most appropriate only for crisis-oriented situations in which rapid mastery of external situations was required. With increased experience, more ambitious goals have been sought. These include, in addition to symptom relief, regaining a sense of emotional equilibrium, developing enhanced coping skills leading to a greater sense of mastery in social and interpersonal situations, and acquiring greater insight into ways of seeing the self and relationships. The extent of these objectives begins to blur the distinction between supportive therapy that hopes to enhance coping skills and more intrusive techniques that seek to promote greater insight into the connections between internal states and interpersonal behavior (14).

There is essential agreement in the literature concerning basic strategies for both individual and group time-limited psychotherapy. These are elaborated in detail throughout this book, but as an overview include

1. The establishment of a time limit will increase the tempo of work and encourage rapid application to outside life circumstances.
2. Careful assessment and selection is important to rule out patients at risk for harm from an active approach.
3. An explicit agreement regarding circumscribed goals should be negotiated openly with the patient.
4. The therapist should intervene actively to develop a therapeutic group climate and to maintain a working focus on the goals identified.
5. The therapist should encourage application of learning to the present, both within the group and in current outside circumstances.
6. The therapist should encourage and expect patient responsibility for initiating therapy tasks.
7. The therapist should encourage the mobilization of outside resources that will reinforce positive changes.
8. It is anticipated that change will continue after termination as the results of therapy are applied; therefore, all problematic issues do not need to be addressed within the therapy context.

Summary

This review of the historical background of contemporary group psychotherapy has emphasized major trends and used the contributions of selected individuals as examples. The available knowledge from clinical and research efforts suggests that there are multiple therapeutic processes at work in therapy groups. Many of these appear to be generic experiences that are relatively independent of theory and are supplied by most therapists regardless of their therapeutic orientation.

Current approaches to understanding group processes represent a melding of two major traditions, psychoanalytic psychotherapy and social psychology. The task of promoting a therapeutic culture has been superimposed onto the traditional role of interpretations by the leader. This has led to a greater appreciation of the importance of group cohesion and member-to-member learning. In technical terms, this creates the need to consider the relative importance of a "corrective emotional experience" versus the need for development of insight into pathogenic patterns. Both approaches will be addressed in this book.

A further technical question that remains unanswered concerns the importance of genetic interpretations dealing with family-of-origin issues. Groups offer a more varied array of interactional stimuli for learning than individual therapy. Many group therapists favor interpretations directed primarily at these here-and-now process experiences. Another central issue concerns the most effective manner for conceptualizing the whole group. In this book, General Systems Theory terminology is adopted as a way of integrating group and individual levels of conceptualization.

These approaches to time-limited group psychotherapy have developed in the context of a parallel movement in individual psychotherapy. Both modalities share a number of common strategies for dealing with the limitations imposed by a defined time limit.

CHAPTER 2

The Small Group

The material in this chapter is drawn from the social psychology literature dealing with the basic science of group behavior. The psychotherapy literature can be properly criticized for emphasizing abstract theories to the exclusion of simple behavioral phenomena. Often the effects of the group context are neglected in favor of theories that stress individual pathology. This chapter, and indeed most of this first section, attempts to redress that imbalance (15).

One advantage of the social psychology perspective is that it describes groups in nontherapeutic and nonpsychopathologic language. This allows the leader to conceptualize the group as a collection of individuals going through the expected tasks of forming and maintaining a social system. An understanding of normal groups encourages a differentiation between expected group behavior and behavior stemming from maladaptive individual issues. This distinction between levels of conceptualizing behavior is crucial. Chapters 4 and 5 concerning group development and social roles provide examples of looking at behavior from the standpoint of the group. Chapters 6 and 10 consider the individual. Each level needs to be considered separately before making assumptions regarding the meaning of particular behaviors.

This chapter begins with a discussion of the group concepts of cohesion and norms and the effects of group size. This is followed by several topics reflecting the perspective of the individual on the group, dealing particularly with issues that influence cognitive appraisals of the group experience. Finally, the basics of operant conditioning are reviewed as a reminder that these learning mechanisms are actively occurring in groups and can be used to promote therapeutic goals.

Group Cohesion

It might seem easy to identify a group that has a high level of cohesion. Terms like *group spirit, esprit de corps, high morale, commitment, team players*, and *group energy* come to mind. At a personal level, one is attracted to some groups, eager to attend, participate, and be identified with the leader and members. This feeling of "groupness" evokes a basic sense of belonging and acceptance that is above and beyond the relationship with any single member, including the leader. Group cohesion constitutes a fundamental property of therapy groups. It serves to sustain the group through difficult therapeutic work. It is a necessary base on which the therapeutic factors discussed in this chapter are grounded. Some of the markers of a cohesive group include

1. Regular and punctual attendance
2. Few premature terminations
3. No regrets about joining and wanting to remain
4. Attraction and warmth between the members
5. High levels of active participation
6. High levels of self-disclosure and trust
7. High-frequency use of the pronoun *we*
8. Low levels of defensiveness and tension
9. Risk taking regarding new behaviors
10. A shared belief system about the goals and norms
11. An investment in the work of the group
12. An ability to focus the work around a common theme

In short, members of a cohesive group view it as important and right for them. All of these positives do not imply that a cohesive group cannot also be challenging and deal with confrontation and anger. Indeed, the opposite is probably the case. In the cohesive group, negative material can be more readily addressed.

In a highly cohesive group, there are stronger efforts to influence others and a greater susceptibility to be influenced. Members are more willing to listen to what others say about them and to accept feedback from others. Cohesive groups strive to protect group norms and to pressure those who deviate to conform to group expectations. These features raise important questions for the group therapist. What is the optimum balance between group membership and individual autonomy? When is the group influence in a positive direction and when can it exert harmful effects? These sorts of questions will be addressed in later chapters.

Cohesiveness represents a necessary quality for effective group psychotherapy. It is a condition for change. Outcome studies indicate that cohesive groups have fewer dropouts and better results. In Chapters 7 and 8, it is emphasized that the therapist must devote specific attention to the primary task of creating a therapeutic group milieu (16).

Group cohesion is analogous to the "therapeutic alliance," a phenomenon that has been well researched in individual psychotherapy. The patient's view of the alliance is a more accurate predictor of outcome than that of the therapist or an observer. Indeed, a strong early positive alliance is one of the better predictors of eventual outcome, its presence indicating that the tools are in place for effective work. The patient's contribution to the alliance appears to be the more decisive element, given a minimal level of therapist facilitation. The therapeutic alliance can be considered under two related dimensions, the *helping alliance* and the *working alliance*.

The concept of the helping alliance stems from the pioneering work of Frank (1973), who has given eloquent expression to the importance of hope, acceptance, support, and confidence as common factors in all therapies. He saw these qualities as powerful tools to combat a state of demoralization and hopelessness/helplessness. This work is closely tied to the Rogerian therapist dimensions of unconditional positive regard, nonpossessive warmth, genuineness, and accurate empathy. In a therapy group, these same factors are distributed throughout the membership and contribute to the development of cohesion.

The working alliance refers to a process of collaboration between therapist and patient on the work of therapy and the adoption of a mutual frame of reference for understanding behavior. Therapy moves faster and more effectively when therapist and patient share a common set of terms for comprehending difficulties and agree on the basic goals of therapy. Much of the effort of pretherapy preparation for group therapy is devoted to this task. The process of universality during early sessions encourages the formation of a strong working alliance.

The helping and working alliances tend to be highly correlated. However, it is useful to think of the features of each as specific dimensions to be reinforced during early sessions (17).

Group Climate and Norms

It is commonplace to describe a group in general terms: "I enjoy going there because the atmosphere is so friendly." "Be careful in there, they jump on everything you say." "I hate going there, nobody takes any responsibility for making decisions." These statements could be made of any group, be it social, administrative, or therapeutic in nature. Such "social climate" opinions reflect the view of an observer or participant about general interactional tendencies in a group and may be quite idiosyncratic in nature. No two participants may "see" the group in quite the same way.

The nature of the group climate will reflect multiple factors including the setting, the style of leadership, the personalities of the members, and how long the group has been meeting. The interactions shown in a group reflect to some extent the internal expectations the members have about what is appropriate behavior. Thus, group climate is closely related to group norms. The language of group climate will be used in Chapter 4 to track the stages of group development.

Groups can be described using everyday terms, but there is some value in using a standard set of dimensions. Two systems, the Group Environment Scale and the Group Climate Questionnaire, are described in Chapter 16. Group climate is an important way of conceptualizing a group. The manifest behavior shown in a group will have a major impact on what members are likely to do. This includes the likelihood of therapeutic or destructive events occurring. The group climate, like the weather, is continually shifting. The leader must learn to systematically track these changes (18).

Another way of conceptualizing and describing small groups is through the language of group norms. The term *norm* is used in two ways. It may be taken to mean a factual description of what actually happens in a given group. This would be captured by the instruction, "Try to describe, not what should, might, or could occur in this group, but what actually does happen." This approach is represented in studies of group climate.

A second, and more theoretically pure, approach is to define norms as the perception by the individual of what the others in the group think or feel about a given course of action. This implies that norms are a statement of expectation, a prediction of how others will react in the future. Hidden in this definition is the idea of conformity, "I ought to do this because I think you think it would be proper." This underlines the mechanism by which social control is usually exerted. It is dependent on the perception and internal interpretation made by the individual member. This process creates a "presumptive reality" that may or may not be accurate.

One convenient way to think of norms is illustrated in Figure 2-1. This is based on group consensus regarding whether or not the behavior is considered acceptable and whether or not it is expected to occur. Behaviors both acceptable and likely to occur are said to be under positive normative control—they tend to be high-frequency behaviors that deal with important group task dimensions such as self-disclosure, providing support, and showing emotion. Behaviors considered to be both unacceptable and unlikely to occur are under negative control—they are usually low-frequency system maintenance functions such as nonattendance and breaks in confidentiality. Risky behavior is that which is acceptable but not thought likely to occur.

EVALUATION

		Consensus considers acceptable	Consensus considers NOT acceptable
E X P E C T A T I O N	Consensus expects to occur	POSITIVE NORM REGULATION (permissive)	DEVIANT BEHAVIORS
	Consensus expects NOT to occur	RISKY BEHAVIORS	NEGATIVE NORM REGULATION (conformity)

Figure 2-1. Model of norm regulation.

Deviant behavior is that which is unacceptable but is believed likely to occur anyway.

Most studies suggest that there is substantial agreement about what should happen in a therapy group, but considerable apprehension about actually doing it. One value in making normative expectations quite clear is that this encourages members to undertake risky behavior. Once enacted, such behavior moves from the risky box to become positively controlled. Members may bring into therapy groups many suppositions about how one should behave in a group, or in fact in any social setting. New or risky behaviors may be inhibited because of uncertainty about the reception by others. That is one reason why a detailed agenda is provided in Chapter 7 for use as pretherapy preparation material. As the group begins, efforts can be made to make normative expectations explicit through specific verbal encouragement and through therapist modeling (19).

Effects of Group Size

The seemingly simple issue of group size may have important ramifications. By changing the number of participants in a group, there will be predictable alterations in the nature of group interactions. Figure 2-2 illustrates how the number of potential interactions in a

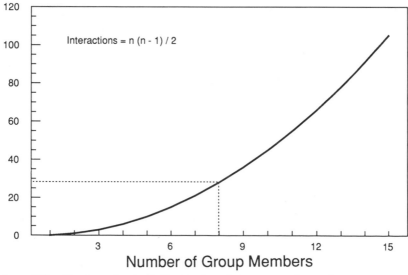

Figure 2-2. Number of potential interactions between members of a group.

group escalates as the number of members increases. This graphically demonstrates that as the size grows, it will become increasingly more difficult to keep track of interaction patterns among the members.

The situation may be even more complex. Often within groups, there are small subgroups of members who identify with each other and are identified as a subgroup by the rest of the members. Such a subgroup may be treated as if it were a separate entity. Two or three subgroups may therefore greatly expand the number of relationship possibilities. To take a common example, a group of eight has the potential of 28 relationship patterns. This would be the case if the group consisted of one leader and seven members. Suppose, however, that the group was actually composed of the same seven members but had two leaders. This simple change of group structure would result in an increase from 28 to 45 possible relationships because each leader could be addressed as an individual or the leaders could be seen as a dyad subsystem.

This simple arithmetic indicates that the size of the group is an important nonspecific variable. In therapy groups, the goal is to help the individual member. This entails an appreciation of how each member interacts with each other member. But how many such patterns can be kept in mind at one time? The leader must select some to follow closely. As the size increases, the percentage to which the leader can attend will progressively decrease. The primary decision about size must therefore be taken quite seriously. It is not a trivial matter to decide to increase the membership from 8 to 12.

As the group size increases, there are a number of predictable consequences:

1. There will be an increased search for leadership, and those with leadership skills will become the focus of group expectations.
2. There will be a greater likelihood of subgrouping, as members seek to satisfy their needs for supportive coalitions and intimacy.
3. Participation rates will become more skewed, as some members dominate the discussion and a larger percentage of members have low rates of activity.
4. There will be more interactions featuring the giving of information or suggestions, and less asking or giving of opinions. This makes the interactional climate safer because the individual risks less.
5. There will be more relationships to maintain and less percentage of time per person to do so.

6. Members will be less inclined to deal with personal matters or take personal responsibility for group direction.
7. Members will pay less attention to their own behavior and how it is perceived by others. In smaller groups, there is greater concern with regulating one's behavior to fit in with the expectations of the group.
8. There will be a greater likelihood that members behave in less inhibited ways with an increase in impulsive behaviors. The possibility of actions that would normally be considered inappropriate by each individual acting alone is increased.

Most of these inevitable consequences of increased numbers work against the promotion of therapeutic work. These interfering effects are counterbalanced by the supportive qualities of a cohesive group environment. In practical terms, group size can be considered as a series of ranges.

Dyads.   Situations involving two people have characteristic interactional features. This is of particular interest to psychotherapists because so much of their work involves a dyadic structure. In comparison with larger groups, tension levels are higher in two-person situations. There is a greater frequency of agreement statements and lower levels of disagreement or antagonism. There is greater likelihood of giving information and asking for opinions, but a lower level of actually giving opinions. These characteristics reflect the need to maintain a delicate balance of power. The participants have only each other to deal with as there is no "public opinion" for appeal or coalition formation. Either member can prevent task accomplishment by disagreement or withdrawal. There is only one person available to respond to distress signals from the other. These interactional challenges are often resolved by the development of asymmetrical roles. One participant assumes an active role of power initiation. The other adopts a passive position with veto power. In this combination, both participants wield considerable influence, though this may not be evident on the surface. It is interesting to apply these characteristics of dyadic communication to the particular circumstances of a psychotherapy session.

Triads.   Groups with three members tend to be preoccupied with alignment issues. To be in a minority position is to be isolated. At any one point in time there is a high likelihood that two members will be paired in competition with the third. This is an unstable pattern, and shifting alliances are common.

Quadrads.   Four-member groups generally find themselves in power contests because of double-pairing phenomena. There is no member to break the impasse, yet each has a source of support. Therefore, deadlocks, phenomena characteristic of all small groups with an even number of members, are common.

Five- to 10-member groups.   Groups with fewer than 5 members spend a lot of energy in coalition negotiations. The result in the case of therapy groups is often a shift toward psychotherapy of the individual in a group setting. From a technical point of view, a group of 5 or 7 members might be considered ideal. This allows each member a subgroup alliance, whereas the uneven number works against polarizations. It is possible to shift roles or positions without forcing a total reorganization of group structure.

Groups of more than 10 members.   Once groups increase beyond 10 members, the complexity of the field gets in the way of attention to the individual. Somewhere around 15–20 members, the possibility of systematic response to individual needs drops sharply, and a classroom atmosphere prevails, which of necessity must be quite leader centered. This may be satisfactory for some types of groups, such as those with a high educational component, but makes individually tailored therapy difficult (20).

Cognitive Mechanisms

Group Interaction Patterns

Groups can be categorized according to their predominant interaction patterns. Figure 2-3 shows several possible patterns in a five-member group. In the wheel diagram, member C is at the center and can interact with all other group members. Each of the other four members interacts only with the person in the center. This puts member C in a position of high control. This pattern is typical of a group conducted by a leader with an active and controlling style. In the circle diagram, all members have equal interaction possibilities, but these are restricted to two members each. This pattern is often found in large groups in which people talk mainly to those seated next to

Network	Adjacency Density	Centrality Index for Position				
		A	B	C	D	E
Wheel 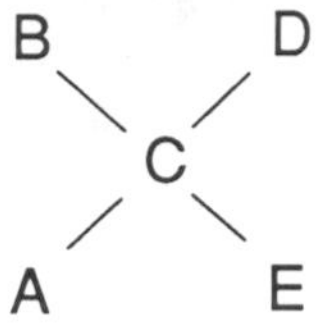	.40	4.6	4.6	8.0	4.6	4.6
Circle 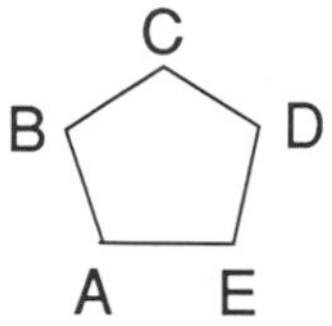	.50	5.0	5.0	5.0	5.0	5.0
Comcon 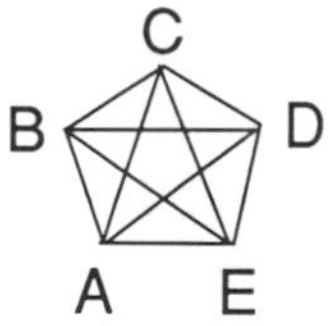	1.00	5.0	5.0	5.0	5.0	5.0

Figure 2-3.   Possible communication networks.

them. In the comcon diagram, the possibilities of interaction are maximized.

An individual member generally reports higher satisfaction with the group experience when his or her own number of possible interactions is high. This is called the *centrality index*, a measure of the degree of communication a given individual has with all other group members. Member C in the wheel diagram has a high centrality index. On the other hand, mean group member satisfaction levels are higher in groups in which most of the members communicate with everyone else. This is termed the *adjacency density*, an index of the overall relatedness links among the members. The comcon pattern achieves a much higher score on adjacency density, with the wheel pattern quite low.

These patterns raise interesting issues for the leader. Does the leader act on behalf of the greatest good for the greatest number and thus strive for the comcon pattern? Does the leader act on behalf of individual members and use a wheel pattern? Some group therapists systematically structure group interaction so that individual members in turn are the focus of attention. When the patterns are totaled for a whole session, the therapist emerges as the central person and therefore has cause to feel most satisfied. On the other hand, perhaps for the individual, the experience of being in the limelight for part of the time counterbalances the lower adjacency density score.

It is useful to think of a group session in terms of such basic communication directionality. Such a perspective may help to identify skewed patterns that have been missed in the heat of a session.

Effect of Social Context on Cognitive Patterns

In social settings, people automatically compare themselves to others, giving rise to "social comparison" theories. This process appears to be an innate predisposition related to basic social functions of acceptance and dominance. In applying this social comparison process, individuals are biased to perceive themselves in a flattering light. At the same time, they are sensitive to the response of others. To varying extents, the self-esteem of the individual is contingent on such responses. People are attracted to groups composed of members who hold generally similar opinions to their own. This makes the process of social comparison easier to understand and anticipate. The person "knows the territory" and can understand the subtleties of the evaluative process.

There is also a tendency for members of a group to see themselves in similar terms. This involves focusing on common issues or characteristics and ignoring or downplaying differences. At the same time, members of a group tend to see the members of other groups in even more homogeneous terms and generally as different in a less favorable direction.

These observations from the literature on small groups have interesting implications for psychotherapy groups. A degree of homogeneity among the members of a group will smooth the development of group cohesion because the members will understand each other more readily and therefore sort out initial social comparison tasks quickly. The therapist can assist this process by actively encouraging members to compare their experiences. Wide extremes in group composition are likely to provoke negative comparative evaluations that may interfere with the development of group cohesion.

Many of the phenomena discussed in Chapter 8 regarding beginning groups demonstrate these early group phenomena. Early in a group's life, there is an "illusion of unanimity" among the members based on unchallenged superficial self-disclosure. These reflexive comparisons are made in the interest of self-validation, not insight, and will occur automatically. In a psychotherapy group in which personal change is the goal, they must at some point give way to more thoughtful consideration.

Another cognitive approach has been developed under the heading of "social cognitive" theory. This perspective is concerned with the manner in which events become symbolic reference points. Social experiences are transformed into enduring internal models that serve as guideposts for future decisions. Possible solutions to present problems can be tested in advance through symbolic planning procedures based on previous events. This implies that present behavior is greatly affected by ideas about its possible future consequences. Through their self-reflective capabilities, people are able to think through future possibilities, test them against personal or vicarious learning, and thus modify their behavior. In a very real sense, the future, or rather our ideas about the future, controls present action. In addition, much of our social learning, to say nothing of specific skills, occurs vicariously through observation, not through trial and error. As the technology of communication advances, for example with television, an even greater portion of our knowledge is gained in this fashion.

A central component to this process is judgments made in regard to one's personal capability to deal with particular situations. This connects directly with Frank's demoralization hypothesis mentioned earlier in this chapter. Most patients present in a state of relative helplessness and hopelessness that is specifically addressed by the cohesive and accepting atmosphere of a group. This work underscores the importance of providing an opportunity for success experiences that enhance a sense of self-efficacy.

This notion of future expectations determining present behavior provides an interesting contrast to the usual psychodynamic perspective that holds present behavior to be heavily influenced by past events. The two viewpoints are not necessarily in opposition because assessments are connected to past experiences. But the therapeutic implications are somewhat different. Cognitive-behavioral techniques stress the importance of understanding the process of distortion in the interpersonal process. Therapy consists of rational attacks on the distorting process. Such an orientation is readily included in group work through the use of "what if" questions. For example, "What do you think would happen if you did tell Elizabeth that she was unfair in criticizing you?" Such techniques combine an understanding of previously learned reactions and future predictions, and application in the present situation (21).

Operant Conditioning

Another perspective on group behavior is provided by learning theory. The principles of operant conditioning are readily apparent in small groups. Positive reinforcers are those that increase the frequency of the target behavior, negative reinforcers decrease it. This does not mean that all positive reinforcers are pleasant. A strong negative reaction to particular behavior may have a powerful positive reinforcing effect. This phenomenon is particularly common with adolescent patients. The wise therapist must be prepared to adopt a neutral stance and assess the actual results of specific interventions. In a group context, the reinforcing messages may come from any or all directions. These effects will be particularly strong in cohesive groups in which there are greater forces to adhere to normative expectations.

The leader is in a place of particular influence to act as an operant conditioner. Groups provide a steady stream of operants—behaviors that operate on the environment—from the members. By attending to these, the leader is in a position to selectively reinforce those behaviors that will enhance the group milieu in a therapeutic direction. Unobtrusive underlining comments will oil the process so that the group can slide smoothly toward its goals. Tiny glissades like "uh-huh," "check that out with him," "that's OK," "say some more about that," and "try that again" serve this purpose.

Throughout this book, specific dimensions or mechanisms by which change can be induced are identified. These phenomena will be evident from the first moment a new group convenes. The therapist can capitalize on these natural processes in order to facilitate the early establishment of a solid sense of groupness by systematically reinforcing appropriate behaviors as they emerge from the membership. By use and reinforcement of this indigenous material, the leader promotes group-initiated patterns that also meet therapeutic requirements. At times it may appear that the group leader is doing very little, but this stance of "masterful inactivity" is a key to successful group work.

Summary

This chapter has drawn material from the social psychology literature. These general ideas about small groups form a backdrop on which therapeutic ideas can be superimposed. The group therapist should appreciate that these general aspects of groupness have a significant impact on the nature of the interactions occurring in a group. It is helpful for the therapist to practice shifting perspective regularly between general group phenomena and individual issues related to psychopathology. At the very least, these ideas may lead to greater enjoyment of administrative meetings, seminar groups, and interactions at the local pub.

CHAPTER **3**

The Group System

This chapter provides an introduction to some basic concepts from General Systems Theory (GST). GST terminology is found increasingly in the group literature because it is well suited to the complexity of groups and the need to consider different levels of organization. A general systems orientation lies behind much of the material in this book. The ideas of norms, therapeutic factors, stages, roles, and recurrent interpersonal patterns are all used in the sense of methods by which the system can become organized (22).

This chapter also describes therapeutic factors that form the mechanisms by which the group experience is helpful. These factors are not tied to a particular theoretical orientation but can be found in varying proportions in all therapy groups. The language in this chapter includes clinical terms like *therapist* and *patient* because the material is derived from experience with groups created for therapeutic purposes.

General Systems Theory

What is a system? The simplest definition is that a system is a structure composed of a whole and its parts. The parts would be useless or helpless without the unifying influence of the whole. The whole is more than the sum of its parts because of the interactive advantages provided by the system. This is sensible enough when considering a watch. It becomes far more complicated when trying to understand a natural ecosystem, an area in which GST had its greatest initial impact.

Living systems take initial internal potential, integrate this with surrounding circumstances, and actively structure their form and organization. The end result of this creative process in any particular situation is difficult to predict. I once had the opportunity of supervising four groups that began simultaneously. As a teaching exercise, about 40 potential members were assigned to groups on the basis of character style, age, and gender so that each group had a rather similar mix. The groups began on the same evening, while I circulated behind the observation windows. Ninety minutes later, four different milieus had emerged, which became increasingly different with each passing session. Despite somewhat similar ingredients, the process of interaction had taken on its own unique quality in each group.

Basic Concepts

One way of conceptualizing this process of development is through the language of GST, with its concern for identifying organizational structures. To begin, here is a brief introduction to some of the basic concepts of GST.

Boundary. This term is not used solely in a physical sense, although it may also represent physical structures, for example, the closed door of the group room. Psychological boundaries exist when there is an awareness that two entities are different; it is this information about differences that constitutes the boundary. For example, the experience of intensive engagement in a group, together with an awareness of how this differs from past interpersonal experiences, begins to establish the external boundary of the group. Throughout later chapters, I use the phrase *boundary massaging* to refer to activities of the therapist that can highlight boundary structures. For example, questions concerning differences across a boundary clarify its very existence. An intervention such as, "You two seem to see the issue differently," leads to increased efforts at clarification of positions and a differentiation process that underscores the boundary.

This process of establishing a boundary provides a mechanism for self-definition. A living cell has an active external membrane that creates a difference in ionic concentrations within the cell as compared with the fluid spaces outside the cell. If the cell pump mechanism fails, the cell dies. In an analogous fashion, a nation creates itself by defining unique internal characteristics through laws and customs and controls these through boundary-crossing procedures. In Chapter 8, the mechanisms by which a therapy group defines itself are discussed.

Opening/closing/permeability.   These are terms that can be applied to boundary functioning. An open boundary encourages acquiring new information, taking risks, and changing. A closed boundary allows reconsolidation of self. Emotion is often thought of as having a powerful boundary-opening effect in human interaction. Thought and language then codify what has happened. Of course, new ideas may also have the potential to induce change. Some types of interpersonal dysfunction can be usefully conceptualized with this boundary language. The obsessive character is notable for relatively impermeable boundaries, whereas the histrionic character may be overly open. Some groups (and families) cannot set external boundaries and are continually besieged by new members, whereas others rigidly maintain membership boundaries and become increasingly isolated. The boundaries most important to group functioning are discussed later in this chapter.

Autonomy.   In a technical sense, this refers to the ability to achieve wholeness, self-regulation, and self-transformation. This process may be understood as the result of external boundary development. Highly enmeshed relationships indicate a lower state of autonomy, with highly permeable boundaries between the participants. A mature psychotherapy group can achieve a quality of autonomy from external issues. It becomes its own world for a time.

Hierarchy.   In complex systems, there are levels of organization. Higher levels integrate the activities of lower levels. The cooperation of two sworn enemies may be explained by their presence on the same team. An important perspective on systems is to understand which level is being addressed. The group diagram later in this chapter embodies the idea of hierarchy. For group purposes, the usual levels to be considered are the group itself, the individual members, and the internal mechanisms for each member. Typically, the group is referred to as the system, and the members as the subsystems. Internal compartments within the individual such as hidden or known psychological issues become the sub-subsystems. Section IV of this book locates the therapy group in the wider suprasystems of a service delivery process and professional disciplines.

Isomorphy.   This refers to the presence of organizing structures that are common across different components of the system. In Chapter 9, parallels are drawn between the individual defense mechanism of projection and the process of scapegoating in a group. Although the nature of the "rejected parts" looks different at each level, they have a common deep structure of projective and displacement mechanisms.

Homeostasis.   This refers to the ability of a system to maintain an internal equilibrium. In groups, social rules and interpersonal feedback loops help to maintain homeostasis. Negative feedback loops maintain the status quo by discouraging behavior outside of expectations. Positive feedback loops encourage novel behavior, risk taking, or experimentation. The idea of stages of group development involves times of change followed by times of consolidation to accommodate to the change.

Specialization.   Components lower in the hierarchy may develop specialized functions that contribute to the higher goals. Behaviors of an individual may seem to make little sense in their own right, but, when considered in terms of the group, the function may become evident. Social roles are one way of describing specialized functions in a group.

Group Structure

A major application of GST to therapy groups consists of the careful understanding of the boundaries that exist in a social system. Figure 3-1 demonstrates a way of diagraming group structure. This format is essentially replicated in the group report form in the Appendix to Chapter 16. The figure is useful for highlighting a series of group boundaries:

1. *External group boundary.*   This involves issues and experiences that create the sense of groupness. These ideas are developed further in Chapter 8 regarding the beginning stages of a group.
2. *Interpersonal boundary.*   It is useful to think of this separately from the individual boundary that defines the individual. The inter-

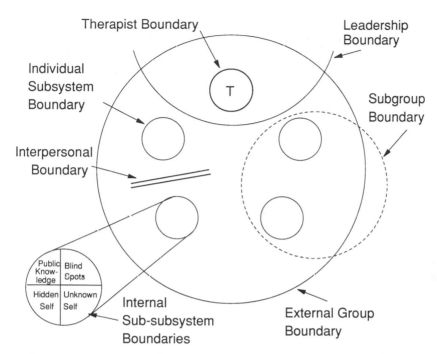

Figure 3-1. Structural diagram of a small group with boundaries identified. Internal structure is based on the Johari Window discussed in Chapter 10.

personal boundary looks at interactions between individuals. In the group of five participants shown in Figure 3-1, there are 10 interpersonal boundaries to consider.

3. *Subgroup boundary.* Frequently, it is useful to think of the group as containing discrete subgroups. These often have fluctuating boundaries. This boundary is shown trailing outside of the group in Figure 3-1, because it may involve issues of extragroup socializing.

4. *Boundary of the leadership subsystem.* The diagram indicates the special importance of the designated leader as a person with extra influence and responsibility. The boundary indicating the leader subsystem may contain a cotherapist and indirectly extends out to include observers and supervisors.

5. *Boundary of the individual subsystem.* This defines information about the individual that is known to others. It represents the individual's sense of self. Some might like to add to this the idea of the social presentation of self, the image we choose to show the world. It is useful to bear in mind that our knowledge of internal processes is dependent on interpretations made from interpersonal

behavior. That is why throughout this book emphasis is placed on the use of interpersonal descriptions before any assumptions are made about internal states.

6. *Boundaries of internal sub-subsystems.*   The language used to describe internal phenomena reflects theoretical orientation. Analysts may use the constructs of superego, ego, and id. Cognitive therapists will describe evaluative mechanisms such as a tendency to be self-critical. One simple but useful way of looking at internal issues is to use the ideas of the Johari Window. This two-by-two matrix is constructed around the categories of information known and not known to self, and information known or not known to others. It is nicely adapted to understanding the process of interpersonal learning as it occurs in groups. These ideas are developed further in the description of critical incidents in Chapter 10.

The schematic depiction in Figure 3-1 captures the idea of a hierarchy of levels for understanding group events. This can be useful as an orienting framework. It does represent an oversimplification, however. For example, the basic assumption states described by Bion are usually thought of as a coming together of relatively primitive response patterns representing internalized object relationship characteristics. These are released from usual control by the environment of the group. Thus, the intrapsychic perspective illuminates the higher-order group characteristics, in a sense reversing the hierarchy (23).

Therapeutic Factors

The therapeutic factors constitute a series of mechanisms that contribute to the therapeutic process. These are described in nontechnical language and have usually been studied by means of patient self-report questionnaires (24).

Group events can be described on a continuum of abstraction. At the most concrete level, the actual behavior occurring in a session can be described or assessed. It is always useful to begin consideration of a clinical event with such basic descriptive information. The assessment of therapeutic factors entails a somewhat greater degree of inference about the meaning of behavior but still lies close to everyday observational data. Ideas about the motivation for or the meaning given to interpersonal behavior move into levels of greater inference where hidden material may play a major role. Intrapsychic concepts such as Oedipal conflict or superego phenomena make major assumptions about internal states that are several steps removed from the behavioral data on which they are based. Each of these levels has its own language and its own justifications. The further one moves from descriptive behavioral language, the more room there is for personal interpretation. This means that there is likely to be less agreement among participants or observers over the meaning of the same event.

Therapeutic factors are viewed as mechanisms generally available within a group and are not specifically linked to therapist actions. Thus, they emphasize group mechanisms over therapeutic strategies. Of course, it is to be expected that each group therapist will influence the mixture of therapeutic factors that emerge, just as group composition will play a part. However, therapeutic factors represent an attempt to describe general group mechanisms inherent in the very fact of an interactional group environment.

The therapeutic factors work in a mutually reinforcing fashion with group cohesion. Enactment of the factors improves cohesion, and a cohesive group promotes the factors. There is value in trying to isolate these individual factor components so that the therapist may specifically attend to their presence and encourage their expression. In Chapter 12, therapist style and technique that enhance the development of a therapeutic milieu are discussed.

The list of therapeutic factors naturally clusters into four general headings: supportive factors, self-revelation factors, learning from others factors, and psychological work factors. There is some modest research evidence to justify this clustering, but it is mainly based on related features and common emergence of factors at different times in a group's life.

Supportive Factors

Supportive factors consist of instillation of hope, acceptance, universality, and altruism. They all promote a sense of belongingness and acceptance and are the group equivalents to the "helping alliance." They are supportive in the technical sense that they assist the patient to regain a sense of mastery. The supportive factors are directly targeted at a sense of demoralization and reduced self-esteem.

Instillation of hope. The idea that there is some chance of relief or improvement is a powerful mechanism for reducing anxiety. This is a global reaction and has little to do with specifics, although the trappings of a therapeutic atmosphere will enhance its development. It is erroneous to call this only a placebo factor. The development of a sense of hope carries with it motivation to engage in therapy, thus providing exposure to other therapeutic factors. A sense of hope will be accompanied by a reduction in anxiety-mediated symptoms that further reinforces motivation to continue.

Instillation of hope is a mechanism common to all therapeutic undertakings. It applies just as strongly to pharmacologic management as it does to psychotherapy. Professionals in training are often reluctant to use techniques that might promote hope, feeling that they are above such common mechanisms that smack of the charlatan or shaman. Indeed, the latter are often more skilled at using this therapeutic factor than professionals. Before an assessment interview ends, it is useful to make some comments to the effect that you are pleased the patient has sought consultation because you believe that something useful can be done.

Acceptance.   In individual therapy, acceptance is a given. There is a general expectation that the healing role will encompass an attitude of basic good will and concern. The situation in a psychotherapy group is different. Acceptance by other members is not automatic and to some extent must be earned. Once achieved, however, the feeling of acceptance and belonging is highly self-enhancing. Because most patients coming for therapy are to some extent struggling with problems of self-esteem, the experience of acceptance is specifically helpful. It counterbalances a sense of shame that may accompany the acknowledgment of the need for help. A patient has to try very hard to be unpopular in the early stages of a group, and the process of acceptance usually develops quickly. It is for this reason that it is important for each member to participate verbally in the first session. This allows an opportunity of response from other members that implicitly acknowledges acceptance.

Universality.   A related therapeutic factor is that of universality, an understanding that others have experienced similar events, thoughts, or reactions. This process is not confined to therapy groups. Early conversation at a cocktail party often involves questions designed to establish common ties: "I lived in Dallas once (before the crash)," "Have you ever been interested in squash," and so on. By finding threads of common experience, people are pulled together and have a way for beginning to associate. In addition, some commonality implies that the other is going to be understandable.

This is a particularly powerful mechanism early in the group. Many people come to group psychotherapy with experiences of loss, disappointment, or guilt. These reactions are often accompanied by the belief that one's situation is unique and that "no one else could ever possibly have experienced such things." To hear that others indeed have shared similar experiences is highly therapeutic. It allows the person to rejoin the human race. Psychological problems frequently lead to increasing social isolation, so that the experience of a boundary-opening exchange is doubly powerful. Issues can be addressed as problems to be solved, not as catastrophes to which one must capitulate. Because of universality, it is possible to generate group discussions in which different reactions to the same type of issue may be discussed. This allows the individual to break out of a restrictive mode of conceptualizing the issue, often one that in the past has precluded successful mastery.

Altruism. Altruism refers to an action that benefits another individual. It is a therapeutic mechanism that is not available in individual psychotherapy. The idea that one can help someone else reinforces self-esteem. It can begin the process of creating a sense of worth and value in one's thoughts or behaviors: "I really appreciated hearing what you said, it helped me to see things differently."

But altruism has effects that go beyond simple kindness. It creates the impression that the giver is a little bit higher on the dominance hierarchy than the one being helped. There is also an implied contract that the favor will be returned at another date. In the primate literature, the term used is *reciprocal altruism*, and it is predicated on the assumption that the two involved animals will have a chance for further activity together so that an opportunity might emerge for the payoff. Altruism is an important mechanism in consolidating social system bonds.

Correlation of supportive factors. The therapeutic factors in this supportive cluster are correlated. People who are altruistically helpful will feel accepted by others. Universality will promote hope. Hope will stimulate participation, which in turn can develop ideas of universality. These supportive factors are particularly critical during the first stage of a group. It is easy to see how they will work together to develop a cohesive atmosphere in which the members feel wanted and accepted. By conceptualizing supportive factors clearly, the therapist can specifically reinforce them and bring them to the awareness of the members. A patient who has fearfully avoided any close relationships may miss statements of acceptance by other group members. The therapist can usefully stop the action and ask for a restatement as well as a response from the fearful patient. In this way, the therapeutic mechanism can be emphasized. New groups will move into statements of universality automatically and quickly. The therapist need only facilitate this by linking statements between members. Situations in which one member offers some assistance to another through support or an explanatory statement may be acknowledged by the therapist or a response prompted from the recipient.

These four therapeutic factors are easy to recognize in group interaction once one thinks of them. Although it is true that they are particularly helpful during the opening stage of a group, they continue to function as important sustaining factors throughout the group's life. When the group is experiencing stress, conflict, or membership change, it is useful for the therapist to refer back to these factors and once again specifically promote their activity. This cluster of therapeutic factors promotes the development of a helping group atmosphere that will encourage therapeutic work. At the same time, these dimensions, in and of themselves, have an effect on demoralization and help the patient to regain a sense of self-confidence and self-efficacy that will enhance problem-solving capability.

Self-revelation Factors

Self-disclosure and catharsis are two factors referring to factual and emotional self-revelation, respectively. Although they often occur together, this is not necessarily the case, and it is helpful for the therapist to consider each as a specific therapeutic factor.

Self-disclosure. At a pragmatic level, the initiation of the group process depends on some degree of self-disclosure. Pretherapy preparation regarding the importance of talking about personal issues therefore has a major payoff in early sessions. The process of self-disclosing facilitates the enactment of other therapeutic factors, particularly from the supportive cluster, as well as initiating the process of interpersonal learning.

Self-disclosure also places issues "on the table" to be looked at more objectively both by the individual and in the interaction with other group members. Psychological distress is often associated with an inability to "get outside of oneself" and look at problems with some degree of objectivity. Instead, the person remains locked in a state of suspension, feeling that no solution is possible. Therefore, the process of self-disclosure is an important early step in beginning to address personal problems.

Self-disclosure has another effect. By deciding to put distressing information into words, the individual is also enacting a decision to take issues seriously. Many patients come to therapy with an idea of the general direction in which their problems lie, but have not been able to come to the point of addressing them. Indeed, the decision to make an initial appointment represents a movement to take oneself seriously. By putting issues into words, there is a tacit acknowledgment that they must be addressed. The self-disclosing process is evidence of increasing commitment to therapy.

Catharsis.   Catharsis refers to the expression of deeply felt emotion. In a formal sense, this can be considered to be content free, though of course some content is inevitable. From the standpoint of catharsis as a therapeutic factor, the importance lies in getting the emotion out, not simply revealing information. This ventilation process relieves built-up pressure and has a calming effect. A normal grief reaction relies heavily on this mechanism.

The research literature supports the idea that a state of heightened emotional arousal promotes change. At the same time, affective discharge without the chance for cognitive integration is not as effective and may be harmful. Thus, a middle ground can be justified where emotional self-revelation is encouraged but reflection on the material is also expected. Therapy that is highly cerebral is probably avoiding important affective material. Therapy that is all emotional may be avoiding an integration and reconciliation of the issues. In terms of boundaries, affect opens the individual boundary and allows a shift in perspective, thinking about the experience gives structure and meaning.

The two self-revelation categories often occur together, but they may appear in a differentiated fashion. Both reflect willingness to be open to others in the group and to sensitive personal material whether it be of a cognitive or emotional nature. The simple process of self-revelation is in itself quite anxiety reducing. The presence of others appears to enhance the effect of catharsis. Self-revelation usually triggers a series of other helpful interactional events.

Learning From Others

These factors include modeling, vicarious learning, guidance, and education. To therapists who value either high affective discharge or deep insightful revelations, these four factors may seem pallid and weak. However, they are reported surprisingly often by group members as being important to their therapeutic progress.

Modeling.   Copying what others do is a major learning strategy. The model provides a message of permission and safety, as well as specific skills. Because modeling will inevitably take place, the therapist can purposefully demonstrate interpersonal dimensions such as support or clarification. This may be done quite openly with the suggestion that members try the same techniques. Similarly, when a group member models therapeutic behavior, its nature can be made explicit. Care must be taken that this process does not have an undesirable effect of appearing to reward favorites.

Vicarious learning.   This refers to a process related to modeling in which members observe interaction among other group members, consider the issues, and then privately apply them to their own circumstances. A major theory in Greek drama, to which group psychotherapy is a close relation, was based on the idea of vicarious emotional learning through the figures on the stage. Because this mechanism is so pervasive, the therapist may promote it by using questions such as, "What were people able to learn from seeing these two have this discussion?" or "Have any of you thought how you might apply these ideas to your situations at home?" This promotes an attitude of constant learning from group interaction. By bringing the issues into awareness, there is also a greater likelihood that they may be tried out in the group, thus adding an experiential component to the learning process.

Guidance.   There are many opportunities during group interaction for advice or guidance to be given. This is particularly common in early groups when there is not yet a climate in which issues are spontaneously explored. Advice may present the individual with options that had not before been considered. Sometimes, practical advice serves to break through resistance when fancy interpretations are rejected. Advice giving may also contribute to altruistic experiences.

It is inevitable that advice and guidance will take place in a group, but the therapist needs to be alert to the potential inhibiting effects of advice giving. Guidance implicitly is a statement of control ("I believe that you should do such and such") and therefore to some extent inhibits member autonomy. Advice offered only as a suggestion to be considered allows room for acceptance or alteration. Advice given to set up a new type of behavior to counterbalance destructive behavior may be useful. Groups that are designed for supportive work on specific problems may use guidance frequently, as will groups operating under behavioral or cognitive-behavioral principles. If the goal of the group is self-exploration and increased autonomy, then advice and guidance should be at a lower level. On the other hand, many patients report that simple instructions to stop destructive behavior or to follow through on socially appropriate action have been quite helpful in moving them through a phase of resistance. Cognitive-behavioral therapy stresses patterns of thinking—the manner in which an individual structures his or her experiences. This approach has had its greatest application in the treatment of depression and phobias. The techniques make full use of guidance, the therapeutic focus on the present and future, not the past. Cognitive techniques are designed to identify, test, and modify distorted conceptualizations and the dysfunctional beliefs (schemata) underlying them. This statement could equally be applied to the idea of psychodynamic insight, although the language used might be different. There is a general trend toward the integration of techniques, and the group therapist can be alert to opportunities to introduce cognitive-behavioral strategies.

Education.   Some forms of group therapy use didactic educational principles. For example, brief groups for patients with bulimia are often structured around specific health topics. Experience suggests that these provide a useful function for many patients and provide an opportunity to select those who require more intensive psychotherapeutic work. The role of education in psychotherapy groups is often neglected. Yet patients who complete treatment are in many respects "experts" in how groups function and in the application of psychological principles. The acquisition of this knowledge can be handled as an overt process. Indeed, a learning paradigm is quite appropriate to the idea of psychotherapy. The language of education—*learning, new ways of understanding,* and *homework*—can add to the therapeutic experience and frame it in a positive direction of mastery rather than a negative orientation of deficit.

The learning-from-others factors are not generally emphasized in psychodynamic circles. However, they certainly occur with great regularity, even in groups supposedly run along nondirective lines. The therapist needs to be alert to their presence to ensure that they are being used in a constructive fashion.

Psychological Work Factors

Self-understanding and interpersonal learning are two therapeutic factors concerned with the acquisition of insight into one's behavior or reactions and learning from interactional events. These two processes are difficult to separate because they represent the internal and external components of the same process. Insight focuses on internal states of mind that are revealed in interpersonal action. Interpersonal learning results in enduring internal alterations concerning how the individual views the interpersonal world. Interpersonal learning has been divided into input and output categories. Input refers to the effects of receiving feedback from others. Output concerns attempts to try out new behaviors with others. Self-understanding can be viewed as the resulting "corrective emotional experience." Compared with individual therapy, the tempo of interpersonal learning is generally more vigorous, multifaceted, and unpredictable in groups. In Chapter 10, the discussion of critical incidents centers around the process of psychological learning. These psychological work factors will be discussed in detail there.

Summary

This chapter has introduced the language of General Systems Theory. The idea of the therapy group as a complex set of interacting members that can be understood at several levels is fundamental to clinical work. The importance of identifying boundaries and using these as a therapeutic focus will be developed in later chapters. Therapeutic factors provide a considerable portion of the help attributed to group therapy. They are understood as mechanisms residing in the very nature of group interaction and are not dependent solely on therapist interventions. A simple clustering of the therapeutic factors described in the literature is provided.

CHAPTER 4

How Groups Develop

This chapter provides an overview of group developmental stages. In Chapter 5, social roles will be described that identify the contribution made by different types of members to the development of the group system. Developmental stages and social roles together constitute a theoretical infrastructure for organizing group phenomena. These two chapters outline the principal ideas in a condensed fashion so that the full range of the material can be surveyed at one time. The material will be applied to clinical work In greater detail in Chapters 8–11.

The Concept of Development

The idea of social systems maturing over time grows out of the general systems orientation introduced in Chapter 3 and the importance of boundaries for defining a system. Development is reflected in the emergence of boundary issues that, if successfully addressed, result in a gradual deepening of the group experience. An appreciation of the group task being addressed in each stage may help the therapist to understand the significance of some types of member behavior.

The phenomenon of developmental stages in groups is found in both the social psychology literature and in studies of clinical groups. Some authors limit their lists of stages to four, whereas others prefer expanded lists of up to nine stages. In this book, six stages are presented: engagement, differentiation, individuation, intimacy, and mutuality, plus termination.

The notion that groups go through a series of predictable developmental stages is somewhat surprising. It is easy to understand the importance of developmental stages in infants because their development is tied to physiological maturation processes. Group development, on the other hand, is dependent on the individual contributions of mature adults. Yet consistently, in psychotherapy groups, administrative committees, community organizations, or athletic teams, the same patterns emerge. Stage concepts may also be applied to the process by which the relationship between two people deepens over time, as in a marriage or in individual psychotherapy. An understanding of the developmental context gives the clinician a useful perspective on the meaning of social behavior.

The concept of group development is another way of addressing group-as-a-whole phenomena. In Chapter 1, reference was made to Bion's ideas about "basic assumption" states and Whitaker's description of psychological conflict held in common by the group members. These same events can be interpreted in terms of group developmental tasks. As in the individual psychotherapy literature, different theoretical traditions use different metaphors to describe similar events. The language of stage development is a particularly useful metaphor for understanding the group as a whole.

The usual approach to stages is descriptive in nature. In this chapter, stage descriptions are augmented with ideas about the tasks that the group members must address in each stage. This expanded view provides the therapist with pragmatic guidelines regarding the sorts of interventions that might be most useful. In the stage model, group development is conceptualized as an epigenetic process in which adequate resolution of any one stage is in part dependent on satisfactory mastery of the preceding stage or stages. At the same time, the tasks of all stages are continually before the group. For example, the engagement task of stage 1 may come into focus again whenever group membership changes, or whenever the group becomes disillusioned with its progress. As a group develops over time, the members interact with increasing complexity.

The ideas of group development are particularly appropriate for time-limited groups. Because such groups generally have consistent membership, there is an opportunity to observe developmental features more acutely than in groups in which members change. When there are time constraints, groups must move as rapidly as possible into more advanced working stages. By accurately attending to the tasks of stages 1 and 2, the therapist can achieve more time for such work. The more the group experience is packaged into a time-limited format with consistent membership, the more evident will be the progression through stage tasks.

Each group developmental stage is characterized by its own style of internal organization. This may be understood as a task that involves a particular set of interpersonal issues that come into focus during that stage. The task polarizes the members along its particular dimension and implicitly demands that each member reveal a position on the relevant issues. A dialectical tension thus is set up within the group membership that creates a pressure to resolve the extreme positions.

The group task is mirrored within the individual member in whom it will be addressed with more or less ease according to characterologic structure. Each member must participate in attempts to master the task of each stage. Only in this fashion can the members benefit maximally from the group process. Conversely, the process of addressing a sequence of common tasks contributes to a sense of "groupness." Members seriously out of step with the main body of the group are liable to feel alienated. If they are ahead of the majority, they may feel that they are getting little out of the experience. If they are behind, they may experience a drop in self-esteem because of their failure to participate with the other members. In time-limited groups, this is a strong argument for a certain degree of homogeneity in group composition.

A period of developmental change tends to be followed by a consolidation phase during which the members work out their reaction to the new set of role expectations. Thus, the group structure undergoes a series of transformations, with periods of change alternating with times of consistency. Within each stage, the individual member is forced to confront the issues "in focus" during that stage. The stage tasks encompass the major themes of human development. They form a predictable sequence by which human relationships are deepened and enriched. In relationships, as in individual growth and development, one must learn to walk before learning to run. The times of transition between stages are critical points of change during which new and more complex interactional behaviors are attempted by group members (25).

Developmental Stages

Stage 1: Engagement

The first task of the group is to ensure that all members are engaged in its activities. If the group does not coalesce, then "group therapy" cannot occur. This process entails a commitment from each member to participate. The interpersonal dimension that becomes polarized in stage 1 is along an axis from trusting and relying on the group at one end, to keeping separate and distant on the other. The task is addressed through two major mechanisms. The first is the comparison of similarities between the members that promotes universality. The second focuses on the identification of differences between experiences in the group and outside circumstances. This assists in developing the external boundary of the group.

The structure of the group is portrayed in Figure 4-1. The boundary focus is on the external boundary of the group. This underscores the need for group identity and definition. The designated leader is the only person about whom the group members have some knowledge and some specific expectations. The leader created the group, selected the members, and signals the beginning by closing the door of

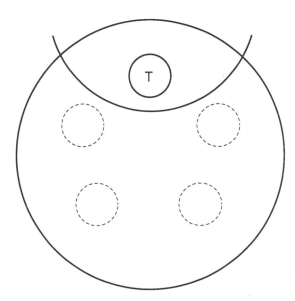

Figure 4-1. Group structure in the engagement stage.

the group room for the first session. The members do not yet represent real identities; they form an undifferentiated membership cluster.

The task for individual members is to allow themselves to become part of the group. Almost everyone experiences anxiety when faced with the task of entering a new social system. Often this fear is associated with the idea that one will not fit in, will be found different, and perhaps will be asked to leave. The task of "getting in" the group is usually handled by self-disclosure. The tentative and partial nature of these self-disclosures is paralleled by the tendency for the other group members to accept them in an uncritical fashion. Members will actively seek positive identifications and similarities rather than make critical or negative critical comparisons.

The process of self-disclosure and the resulting sense of acceptance is of far greater importance during the early stages of a group than the actual content discussed. When individuals put into words the concerns they hold about themselves, they are implicitly acknowledging the need to work on these issues; that is, they are accepting themselves as objects of concern. This process of acknowledgment is the first major step toward successful therapy. The identification of goals with some commonality to other members enhances the universality experience. All of these experiences serve to differentiate the group experience from outside circumstances. They create a sense of what this particular group is going to be about.

The tasks of the engagement stage can be considered accomplished when all members have actively participated in the group and there is a rising sense of satisfaction and commitment to participation. There is a conviction that the group is going to survive and a comfortable sense of cohesion. This is very similar to descriptions in the individual psychotherapy literature of a positive working alliance. Groups may become stuck in the relatively pleasant but non-challenging atmosphere of the first stage, and the leader must be prepared to assist the group in moving on once the stage tasks have been accomplished.

Stage 2: Differentiation

The central tasks of the second stage of group development are to recognize that differences exist among members and to develop methods for conflict resolution. The term *differentiation* identifies the tasks of the stage more accurately than the usual descriptive title of *conflict* stage. The work of this stage contrasts with the focus on similarities in the first stage, and the emergence of this thematic shift is inherently more difficult and anxiety inducing. However, a more confrontational style addresses the tendency in stage 1 to show uncritical acceptance. A cooperative style of addressing differences must be developed.

The interpersonal axis being examined in this stage lies between the active initiating pole of confronting and asserting, and the avoidance of conflict through passive acceptance. This is a shift from stage 1, in which most of the behaviors lay in the positive and reacting spectrum.

The new group structure is portrayed in Figure 4-2. The focus is now on the individual boundary of each member. This produces friction at the interface with others, but the task of the group is focused on recognizing the individual. "Real" identifiable people are beginning to emerge, though they are still seen in rather general and somewhat stereotypic terms. The designated leader still plays a predominant role in the group.

The process of interpersonal challenge that is going on at the group level will be echoed at an internal level for each member. The need to justify one's position through assertive statements forces increased self-disclosure. The process of defending oneself, taking stands, and criticizing others will often bring to the surface aspects of

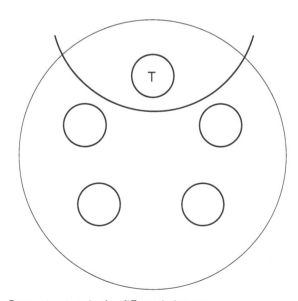

Figure 4-2.   Group structure in the differentiation stage.

the self that are viewed ambivalently or negatively. These self-percepts may be as polarized as those within the group generally. Often they are seen as autonomous urges or mysterious reactions beyond conscious control: "The Devil made me do it." Indeed, the exaggerated and stereotypic aspects of the group process in stage 2 often entail the use of projective defenses through which rejected aspects of self are reacted to in others. The group process helps the individual to acknowledge personal issues that need to be addressed. By putting these into words for the group, the member is at the same time clarifying them for self. The individual must become able to tolerate reactions of anger and conflict in self and others. These may be associated with the fear of destructive loss of control.

The individual is also challenged by the group to conform to explicitly stated group expectations. This entails a greater commitment to groupness, which may be interpreted as a loss of individuality. The process of working through these issues serves to consolidate group cohesion and engenders a deeper commitment to the group by its members. The stage reaches its closure when all members have participated to some extent in the assertive work of self-expression and when the group is able to tolerate challenges and confrontations as constructive events. The members realize that they are acceptable to the group even when they seem to be at their worst. There is a recognition that everyone does not need to have the same viewpoint in order to get along. Stage 2 often ends unexpectedly. The leader may come out of one session fearing that the group is going to self-destruct and enter the next session to find a happily interacting working group.

The group moves on from the first two stages with two important qualities: a sense of universality regarding common problems and goals and an ability to tolerate differences and challenge them. Important work has been done on two major aspects of interpersonal functioning—affiliation tasks in stage 1 and self-definition tasks in stage 2. Thus, the first two stages of the group equip the system for more complex interpersonal work. The interactional milieu is becoming more complicated as the system continues its process of maturation.

Stage 3: Individuation

The task of the third stage is to promote an exploration of the diversity within each member. In stage 2, we saw the beginning of the emergence of self-definition. In stage 3, this process continues with efforts to understand the complexity of the individual. Although this process is conducted through interpersonal dialogue, the content emphasis is on the individual more than on the interaction between individuals (26).

The internal focus calls for an attitude of openness to psychological issues and the relinquishment of a defensive posture. This work polarizes for each member an introspective attitude toward self that has self-blaming and self-oppressing qualities at one end, and self-accepting and self-exploring qualities at the other.

The schematic diagram of the group now undergoes a major shift (Figure 4-3). The designated leader is no longer the center of group attention. The individual members have emerged as fully identifiable individuals. The boundary area in focus has to do with internal issues for each member. This stage is characterized by a marked increase in knowledge about how one functions psychologically. Hidden or unacknowledged material is brought under greater scrutiny.

The central task for the individual member is to challenge characteristic defensive mechanisms. This attention to personal motivations and the consequent interpersonal implications of them allows the individual to view private issues more objectively. In this process, the individual may face a serious threat to self-esteem as previously unacknowledged parts of self are explored. In the longer term, it usually stimulates an expanded view that reinforces self-image.

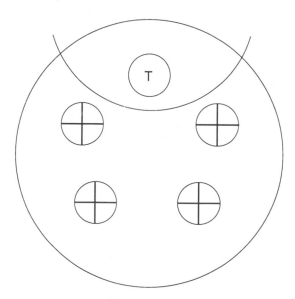

Figure 4-3.   Group structure in the individuation stage.

The work of the third stage produces a great deal of personalized information about each member. Participation in this process draws the members closer together, and group cohesion and morale are generally high. The shift to stage 4 is often heralded by the introduction of topics related to close personal relationships. This is a natural progression that uses the knowledge and closeness gained in stage 3.

From this point on in the life of the group, the transition between stages becomes less obvious. Some authors have been content with describing only three stages of development before termination, leaving everything after the conflict stage in one large working category. However, even though the transition zones may be less precise, there is value in considering two further working stages that entail consideration of two basic axes of social life, intimacy, and autonomy. In a sense, this sequence represents a reworking of issues that were first addressed in stages 1 and 2. Engagement is deepened by addressing intimacy issues, and the differentiation task moves into issues of autonomy in relationships. This idea of a deepening spiral of recurring work themes captures an important aspect of group development.

Stage 4: Intimacy

The central task in this stage is to come to terms with the increasing closeness that develops among the members as the group matures. In a technical sense, the increased information that the members now have about each other draws them into closer here-and-now interaction. As greater familiarity develops, the individual members have greater influence on each other and may experience levels of intimacy sometimes greater than any they have found elsewhere in their adult lives. This entails acknowledgment that the acquaintanceships of stage 1 have developed into real relationships. Relationships between members have now begun to replace the relationship with the leader as the principal concern of the members. This task will polarize the members along an "affiliation" dimension. At the positive end, this reflects warmth and closeness toward others. At the other end, rejecting or isolating reactions indicate problems with the affiliation process.

The boundary focus is now primarily at the interface between individual members (Figure 4-4). Special relationship subgroups may develop. The boundary for these is shown as extending outside the external group boundary because there is greater likelihood of extragroup socializing during this stage.

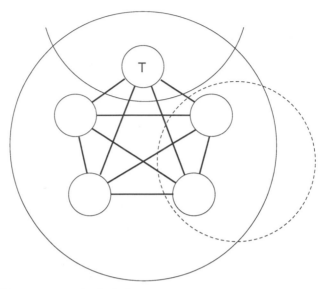

Figure 4-4.   Group structure in the intimacy stage.

The work of this stage provides an opportunity to explore the importance of relationships. This will bring with it the threat of rejection by persons who have become known in a highly personalized fashion. Because this is a common problem with patients seeking psychotherapy, the opportunity to explore these reactions provides a powerful experience. This entails an acceptance of self as capable and worthy of closeness and a dimension of trust that the other will tolerate this and reciprocate. This work addresses the universal human need for closeness and acceptance.

The work of stage 4 is generally conducted in a positive atmosphere, sometimes reminiscent of the euphoria of stage 1. There is an excitement in the air. Consistent attention to the task will lead to sobering second thoughts concerning the responsibility of intimacy. This gradual shift leads into the work of stage 5.

Stage 5: Mutuality

The task in the fifth stage is to explore the responsibilities of close relationships. This concerns an appreciation of the fundamental uniqueness of each member and the balance between individual autonomy and interpersonal involvement. The members become aware that mature relationships cannot be determined unilaterally by one person but must be based on an interactive process of mutual agreement and consent.

The work of this stage is polarized along the independence/ interdependence axis. At one end, this entails a consideration of unbalanced relationships based on dependency or control that are quite enmeshed. The other extreme goes beyond the recognition of independence from the other to a degree of separateness that leads to isolation.

The schematic group diagram now achieves its most complex structure with strengthened interactions among all members (Figure 4-5). The focus remains on interpersonal relationships, but the boundary of the individual member is now highlighted. The subgrouping typical of stage 4 is less evident.

The mutuality stage addresses questions of irresponsible closeness that were raised in the preceding intimacy stage. Questions of dominance or submission in relationships are explored. The task of accepting responsibility for one's interactions with others as equals involves working at a high level of personal maturity. Issues of trust often come into focus during this process.

Members report significantly greater ease in addressing interpersonal issues in the group, and there is more evidence of successful application to outside relationships and circumstances. Questions be-

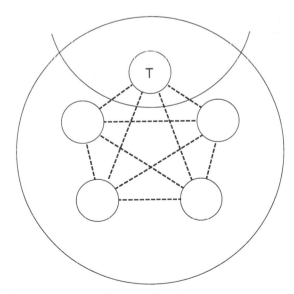

Figure 4-5. Group structure in the mutuality stage.

gin to be raised about how much more therapy is required. Other personal projects and ambitions begin to intrude on the insularity of the room. Attention is again being directed to the external group border.

Termination

The final stage in the life of a group is its ending. No number is given to this stage because termination may occur at any time depending on the duration of the group, the capacity of the members, and the time available. Whenever it does occur, a common set of issues must be addressed. The central task for the termination stage is to achieve a comfortable sense of disengagement from the group system while incorporating the group events as a positive and constructive experience.

The end of a group means the dissolution of group structural features. We are left with individuals only (Figure 4-6). Within each individual is a memory of group experiences.

The individual member must deal with themes related to loss. Components of sadness and grief are usually contained in these associations, along with disappointment and perhaps anger. Working through of these issues in terms of the group itself and its individual members constitutes necessary termination work. The danger is that the end of the group will be interpreted as abandonment before full recovery has been achieved, which may result in a demoralized state that will lead to an enduring interpretation of the therapeutic experience in negative terms.

As in all stages, the work must be done by each member. A

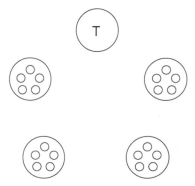

Figure 4-6.   Group structure in the termination stage.

particular problem at the end is that some members may attempt to avoid this task by terminating early or missing final sessions. The therapist needs to participate in this stage as much as the members. The natural sense that more could have been accomplished can be offset with the realization that outcome studies indicate that improvement continues to increase for some time after the actual termination.

Summary

This chapter has summarized a theory of group development. Each stage presents specific challenges and tasks to the group and to the individual member. Stage recognition is most useful as the group is beginning. During stages 1 and 2, the leader's principal responsibility is to assist in the creation of a therapeutic group climate. Once this is achieved, more attention can be paid to individual issues.

The thematic shift between stages usually occurs gradually. Early hints of dissatisfaction with the current level of work may surface, or new behaviors may be briefly tried out in the group. Sometimes stage shifts are heralded by a change in the content focus as outside experiences are described. For example, the onset of the intimacy stage often begins with attention to outside romantic relationships. The therapist should be alert to these hints of change. Through reinforcement of them, the stage transition can be facilitated. The therapist cannot, however, force the group through stages. Blocks or resistances can be addressed so that the members may begin to think of new possibilities in their manner of relating. Stage mastery is assisted by encouraging discussion of the process of, and reactions to, addressing the tasks of each stage.

Therapists may also block group development by discouraging the emergence of behaviors or themes that would lead to the exploration of new material. This may be done purposefully. For example, a brief inpatient group with severely disturbed patients is best kept to an engagement stage of interaction because the circumstances make it unlikely that there will be an opportunity to deal with more intense issues. The therapist may assist in holding the group to this task by emphasizing positive and constructive general discussions and deflecting themes of conflict or confrontation. An awareness of group developmental stages prepares the therapist to make such decisions knowledgeably.

One warning is in order: the idea of group stages, like that of individual growth and development, is a general theory. Individual groups will show unique responses to these general tasks. The ideas contained in this chapter should help to sensitize the therapist to the important issues. Later chapters will discuss in more detail how the therapist may assist the group in mastering stage tasks. At any point, critical incidents may need to be addressed. Specific needs of a particular member may require interventions even if out of harmony with group needs. General clinical skills in psychotherapeutic management are therefore necessary. The group developmental theory is designed as an orienting perspective that can assist the therapist in understanding the relative significance of group events. This provides the leader with guidelines regarding the type of intervention that will be most relevant to the members' experience. For example, issues of an introspective nature may appear in an early session, but to pursue these with zeal may mean that essential group consolidation tasks are avoided.

Group stages are observed most clearly in time-limited closed groups. Such a context provides the maximum opportunity to see a social system develop increasing complexity. In later chapters, the language of group development will be applied in identifying group regression and in appreciating the issues involved at times of group membership change.

CHAPTER 5

Social Roles

The idea of social role connects the interactional style of the individual with the functional needs of the group. The concepts of social role complement the theory of group developmental stages discussed in the preceding chapter. Stages describe the group as an evolving system, whereas roles focus on the impact that types of member behavior have on that system. In Chapter 6, assessment methods will be presented that link the individual patient to these ideas of group organization.

The Concept of Social Role

Social role refers to a group function, not an individual quality. The family literature provides a useful approach to this idea. *Family role position* describes some functional requirement of the family. For example, the family role position of "father" is required. In a single-parent family, this role may be filled by the mother, a male relative, or a boyfriend. The critical point is that the organizational position be filled. Similarly, families can be considered in terms of the parental role system, the spousal roles, or the dependent child role. These concepts may also be applied to group social roles. This matching of group need with individual predisposition makes the idea of social role particularly interesting from a theoretical perspective (27).

One characteristic of patients with neurotic or characterologic problems is a lack of flexibility in their interpersonal relationships. They tend to react in the same fashion in different circumstances, and thus a style that may have been of advantage in one situation becomes a liability in others. A preponderant and overly intrusive interactional style fits nicely with the idea of social role. Indeed, one acceptable definition of therapeutic progress is the development of role flexibility. One implication of this is that a considered effort should be made to provide opportunities for all members to understand and experience the various role behaviors. Thus, the group developmental agenda of increasing complexity of interactional opportunities fits the individual agenda of learning role flexibility.

The Designated Leader

The social psychology literature places great emphasis on the role implications of official leadership. For the clinician, this designation brings with it a host of expectations that provide both opportunities and problems for effective therapeutic work.

Designation as therapist of a psychotherapy group automatically places one in the sociocultural role of "healer." This position carries with it expectations regarding ethical standards as well as appropriate knowledge and skills. It brings expectations that the leader will be helpful and positively motivated toward the members and will assume responsibility for preventing damaging experiences. Chapters 12 and 13 expand on these issues.

In the group structural diagram in Chapter 3, a boundary line was drawn between the therapist subsystem and the other group members. The "differences across the boundary" that form this boundary are heavily influenced by social role expectations. These expectations may have little to do with the actual person or the behavior of the leader. Every group leader (or committee chair) has been amazed at the powerful reactions elicited simply because of sitting in the leader's chair. The image of the "throne" produces strong reactions in both positive and negative directions.

Group therapists are often concerned about the question of responsibility for initiating group activity. Patients will come with the plausible statement, "Since you are the leader, lead us." This is a role expectation trap that requires adroit management. The optimal degree of leader control is related to the goals of the group and to the capabilities of the members, as discussed in Chapter 12.

The review of group developmental ideas in the preceding chapter suggested that a certain amount of therapist initiation is appropriate in the early stages of group. During the engagement stage, the therapist has a responsibility to promote the development of an effective and cohesive system. This responsibility must then be tapered so that the members may feel confident of initiating leadership challenge during the differentiation stage. The process may be assisted through systematic pretherapy preparation, as discussed in Chapter 7, and by continual reinforcement of patient initiative during the early sessions. One therapist goal is the development of a working group that will assume much of the leadership function for promoting therapeutic change. This theme of the therapist using the group as the agent of change runs through much of this book.

At the same time, there are distinct powers given to the designated leader that should not be neglected. By virtue of the role, the leader is in a position to influence group events. Usually this can be done with subtle reinforcement, but if necessary a firm management stance can be taken. The leader is in a position to view group events from the perspective of stage-appropriate challenges and anxieties as well as to conceptualize longer-term change effects. An understanding and accepting therapist who can tolerate group events without overt anxiety exerts an enormously stabilizing effect on the group and allows it to proceed with its work. The role of designated leader will stimulate responses from members that are characteristic of their relationship with parental and authority figures. Material directed specifically to the leader needs to be considered as a special and powerful class of interactional events within the group. It may offer unique opportunities for therapeutic insight. It is a technical challenge for the therapist to encourage the use of this material without at the same time downplaying or deflecting from the learning that can occur through member-to-member interaction.

There is some diversity of opinion regarding how to best respond to reactions to the leader that are above and beyond the real relationship—reactions influenced by the role of designated leader. Some therapists view the group as a setting in which most, if not all, member behavior should be understood in terms of its relationship to the leader. Such therapists spend much time interpreting parental/authority themes. Other group therapists view the group in a more egalitarian light and downplay the prominence of the therapist, while promoting the importance of member interactions. The implications of these positions are addressed in Chapters 12 and 13. In all cases, the role of designated leader must be treated with care and with thoughtful attention to its implications.

Group Social Roles

The majority of studies concerning group roles come not from the psychotherapeutic literature but from social psychology studies, most of which are based on groups that have clearly defined short-term tasks such as solving complex mathematical or administrative problems. The task focus of these studies makes for an uneasy translation into the context of therapy groups, in which the task is of a reflective nature—to study the process of the group and the part each member plays in it. Nevertheless, there are some useful applications of role ideas for the clinician.

Social roles provide a structure for considering the functions of different styles of behavior in a group setting. Social roles constitute one application of characterologic style. Role definitions describe the manner in which individuals understand the nature of their relationship to the group system. This involves typical interpretations concerning the meaning of group events and subjective internal reactions, as well as characteristic behavioral responses. Thus, social roles encompass cognitive, affective, and behavioral components.

Four social roles are described: the sociable, structural, divergent, and cautionary roles. These may be considered as packages of features that generally are found together. Each member may provide some contribution to the role function, but usually some members stand out as fulfilling role criteria more fully. One interesting exercise is to rank the entire group membership on each role function. One or more members may then qualify as role leaders in one of the four categories described. This ranking approach is a more realistic and helpful approach than insisting that only one person can occupy a particular group role (28).

Roles represent adaptive responses to the stresses and expectations of a social system. The social behavior of the individual may be seen as a calculated method, perhaps beneath conscious awareness, to evoke or provoke satisfying responses from others. These personal needs must be balanced against the capacity of the group to satisfy them, as well as the group need for the contributions of the individual. The actual behavior manifested in the group represents the outcome of these opposing tendencies. This is a modified version of Lewin's field theory and Foulkes' group matrix.

The needs of the group are not simply theoretical abstractions. To function properly, a group must have some members who supply the behavioral input represented by the four social roles. These represent organizational axes critical for group development. At a time of need, there will be an expectancy in the air that someone has to fulfill that particular function. Subtle pressure for response will be exerted on members who seem to best fit these requirements. This is referred to as *role suction*. It can be a very powerful force from which the therapist is not immune. There is an almost palpable presence saying, "Help us get through this situation, we need you, don't abandon us." Note the combination of expectation and guilt induction in this phrase. Those members most characterologically attuned to the message are likely to respond. When the group need is high and the personality of the member is strongly polarized along a particular role dimension, the phenomenon of *role lock* may occur. The individual exaggerates usual behaviors and becomes almost a caricature of self, and the process is strongly reinforced by group response.

The stage ideas in the preceding chapter identify some of the input requirements needed by the group at different times. The connections between stages and roles are summarized at the end of this chapter and applied to clinical work in Section II of this book. The ideas of social roles may also be incorporated into decisions regarding group membership. A general principle elaborated in Chapter 7 concerns the advantages of composing a group to contain a spectrum of interpersonal styles. The following description of four social roles provides one method for approaching that task.

Sociable Role

The sociable role is closely connected to the traditional role of the "socioemotional leader." In studies of task groups, this role is seen as providing a quality that is complementary to the activities of the "task leader." Such groups oscillate between a task focus and a tension-release focus. This is explained as a process of tension buildup through task attention that requires venting through emotional discharge including attention to interpersonal friction. The socioemotional leader mediates these sorts of issues. After this process, the group can return to its task focus. Thus, the two leadership styles combine to promote effective task accomplishment.

Members who adopt the sociable role are characterized by an eagerness to establish positive relationships. They place emphasis on providing support and reassurance. Their gregarious nature promotes a sense of trust. They are concerned that all members be included in the group and that all have a positive experience. This may extend from an eagerness to provide care and concern through attention to instrumental support functions such as room arrangements and providing food or coffee. People functioning in the sociable role emphasize the importance of a positive affiliative tone. They will intervene quickly to dampen negatively tinged interactions. They generally have excellent attendance, and they will become concerned about the absence or nonparticipation of other members.

These role activities are particularly important for the group in the engagement stage. Technically, they serve to open interpersonal boundaries and focus attention on experiences between members inside the group boundary. They help to promote group cohesion and will make the group appear less threatening to apprehensive members. Sociable role members are eager to identify with others and therefore promote universality. Because they tend to be trusting, they are able to model early self-disclosure as a group norm. These members often have a touch of naïveté. They tend to use the defense mechanisms of repression and denial, which allows them to quickly and perhaps unrealistically express hope for the success of the group and the effectiveness of the treatment. The cluster of sociable role behaviors, although particularly important during the formative stages of the group, remain as an important sustaining factor throughout the group's life.

These role behaviors may have an inhibiting effect on further group development. Such members will be particularly concerned at the emergence of anger or confrontation and may try to pull the group back into the safer waters of engagement. The thought of group termination is usually difficult for these members, and they may work to delay such an eventuality.

The sociable role members usually find it relatively easy to enter into the group. Because of their benign approach to others, they elicit positive confirming responses and are popular members. Early in the group's life, they are generally seen in a positive light and appear to have a particularly important role. These processes result in enhanced self-esteem for sociable role members, which may be accompanied by an early reduction in symptoms. Their need to maintain a positive and involved position may make it difficult to deal with issues involving anger or criticism, and they may find the introspective task difficult. As the group develops, their difficulty in moving below surface socialization may lead to criticism from other group members. Sociable role members stand to benefit from the advanced working stages of the group in which their qualities of excessive trust and naïveté may be challenged. On the other hand, these same qualities make it possible for such members to be exploited and used by the group as a vehicle for avoidance, a theme that often runs in their personal lives as well.

Sociable role members tend to become dependent on leaders and align with and support their activities. This makes it difficult for them to deal with leader expectations that they become more independent in their self-exploration and interactional activities.

Structural Role

This role is a modified version of the role of "task leader" described in social psychology studies. Historically, the task leader has generally been the designated leader and the role has been equated with formal leadership functions. The following description de-emphasizes the task focus and instead fits the role into a generalized interactional style.

Members adopting the structural role are concerned with understanding and organizing their experience of the group. This provides a focusing and clarifying quality that enhances group work. The structural role members worry about goal accomplishment and will strive to promote positive group outcomes. They are concerned with form and structure and the proper way to do things. This is best understood in terms of their need to maintain a sense of mastery, not as efforts to control the group, though that may be an unintended result. They emphasize cognitive mechanisms and may perseverate with verbal definitions and explanations, using rationalization and intellectualization defense mechanisms in an obsessive fashion. Their interpersonal skills may lack spontaneity, leading them to adopt a compulsive advice-giving style which reflects their difficulty in establishing empathic bonds. In contrast to the sociable role members, who are highly involved with the experience of the group, the structural role members may adopt a working stance that distances them from some members. They want to be part of the group, but are not sure how to achieve this.

Structural role members provide a cognitive structure for the group in terms of goals and expectations. They promote a closing of interpersonal boundaries, allowing time for integration and under-standing of the experience. They are more comfortable bringing in material from outside the group and help to mediate external bound-ary issues. This provides an important ingredient for the developing group. The use of cognitive and distancing techniques may have a calming effect. Their search for clarity and understanding helps to reduce the ambiguity of the group task. They help the group to contain and master affect by focusing on its origins and functions. They may also be particularly helpful in encouraging the application of group material to outside situations.

The structural role activities provide a positive and comple-mentary component to those of the sociable role members. The socia-ble role members focus on process involvement and affect stimula-tion, whereas the structural role members promote cognitive mastery and organization. Too much structuring may act as an impediment to free-flowing group interaction. This can result in a group atmosphere that resembles a debating society more than an arena for experiential learning. Structural role members may actively work to prevent the emergence of affect in the group and thus deprive the group of the stimulus and drive this can provide.

Structural role members find group participation anxiety produc-ing. Despite this, their motivation to succeed and their search for understanding make them productive group members. They are usu-ally accepted as sensible and helpful participants. This recognition allows them to benefit from the group interaction without raising their defensiveness. Their style allows them to be less influenced by high group affect, and they may be able to counterbalance the possibly destabilizing effects of intense emotion.

Structural role members feel most comfortable when the group has a clearly defined task. Particularly early in the group, they may be active with premature attempts to bring closure to the group discus-sions. They may experience helpless bewilderment at the lack of structure and the emphasis on process exploration that is characteris-tic of therapy groups. Their difficulty in dealing with affective open-ness may make it difficult for them to become involved with the group. This is frequently interpreted by other members as indicating a superior attitude. These responses from others may lead to further isolation.

The concern these members have with achieving results puts them in a position to help with the task activities of the therapist. At the same time, it is easy for this relationship to assume a competitive tone.

Divergent Role

The role of the scapegoat has a lengthy religious and philosophical history. It has been well developed in the family therapy literature. The term *divergent role* has been chosen to highlight the function such members have for a social system.

Divergent role behavior is characterized by impulsivity and an emphasis on differences. These members consistently challenge and question what is going on and usually take viewpoints that are divergent from the others. This forces the group to clarify issues. Often there is an angry and aggressive component to this. These members may belittle or blame others and appear themselves to be chronically dissatisfied. This use of projective defense mechanisms may actively elicit a hostile response from other group members. They are very much involved in the action of the group and are seen as important though not entirely welcome members. Often the issues they raise reflect an intuitive understanding of interpersonal functioning.

These members usually have a high profile in the group and serve to promote interaction. Their activity opens interpersonal boundaries, though sometimes in a negative fashion. They are very much caught up in the process of the group itself. Other members frequently view the divergent role members as blocking group progress, and they may become the repository of much angry and blaming material. Divergent role members play a particularly important part during the differentiation stage of group development. They are able to challenge the group to explore differences and ambiguities, and they force the polarization of discussion. This necessitates the development of conflict resolution mechanisms. The divergent role members provide role models for the expression of anger and confrontation. They tend to be persistent and prevent premature closure on important issues and are particularly sensitive to group resistance. The activity of the divergent role members, although not acknowledged as such by the group, does in fact have a beneficial and stimulating effect.

If these dimensions become overly powerful in the group, cohesion and morale may drop because of irreconcilable competitive impasses. The group may try to use these members as a focus for resistance rather than as a focus for exploring issues. There may be efforts to extrude them as a means of resolving group tensions, the classic function of the scapegoat. Such a development is counterproductive for the group as well as potentially damaging for the divergent role member. If there are unexplored tensions in the group, it is inevitable that other members will come, or be pushed, forward to adopt the divergent role because these functions are necessary to address controversial or conflictual issues.

The high level of activity and the intrusive nature of these members forces them into the social structure of the group. Their energy and commitment to fearless challenge may make them admired and respected. These same characteristics may make it difficult for them to maintain the positive regard of group members, and, therefore, they may become isolated from the support that a group can provide. This can launch a destructive process by which they become group casualties. These members usually lead challenges to the therapist. In this, they provide important leadership for the group. There is a danger that this may escalate into a polarized contest of wills with the leader.

Cautionary Role

The cautionary role is a relative newcomer in the group literature, in which it is sometimes referred to as the "defiant member" because these members appear to be defying the power of the group. The term *cautionary* draws attention to the vulnerability these people experience when faced with the challenge of being in a small group.

Like the structural role members, the members taking on the cautionary role are resistant to involvement in the group process. They are reluctant to reveal personal reactions and defensive about providing personal information. For them, a little participation goes a long way. They view the entire idea of group therapy with substantial distrust. These members stress the importance of autonomy and self-control. Their use of withdrawal and avoidance defense mechanisms causes them to appear uninvolved. Their ambivalence about group participation frequently has an angry quality. The cautionary role members are often silent and may miss early sessions.

These members provide a model for individual autonomy that may act as a useful brake on overly rapid involvement in group consensus. Their activities tend to close interpersonal boundaries, and they prefer to work across the external group boundary. These activities force the group to deal with membership commitment issues. The concerns of these members address the common fear among group members that they will be overwhelmed by the group influence and become out of control. Cautionary role members are able to see group events in the context of outside circumstances and may help in the transfer of learning. They are much less threatened by the idea of group termination and may help to put this in perspective for other members.

The negative and distancing qualities of the cautionary role members make their participation in the group difficult, and they tend to exert an anticohesion influence. Such persons become involved in groups reluctantly and are at risk for premature termination. Their difficulty in using the group may activate dimensions of hopelessness in other members.

Individuals of this nature are able to maintain greater personal stability in the face of social pressures. They provide a model of autonomy and self-reliance that is particularly useful for sociable role members. They may help the group to deal with the exploration of negative themes that others wish to avoid. Members who are strong on this dimension have difficulty with the effective use of group therapy. Their withdrawal and lack of response to others may result in a process of isolation and criticism that may reinforce their already strong belief in the danger of social involvement.

These members commonly align with the therapist more than the group members. This may represent for them a more formal relationship with less threat of personal involvement. As the group progresses, they may negotiate a "special relationship" with the therapist as a condition of continuing participation. For example, there may be an implicit agreement that they do not need to participate as actively. This may be signaled by an exchange of meaningful glances between the cautionary member and the therapist at times of group tension.

Summary

The four social roles described in this chapter represent a shorthand summary of important clusters of interpersonal behaviors. The function that each role has for the group may be superimposed on the group developmental stage concepts of Chapter 4.

Stage 1 is primarily concerned with positive affiliative mechanisms and membership. The work of stage 1 is polarized between the sociable and cautionary role members, who view the group from opposite sides of the external boundary.

Stage 2 features the active recognition of differences and negative affect, yet is still preoccupied with participation issues. The divergent role members drive the work of this stage. The structural role members are able to complement the emotional drive of the divergent members with efforts to understand the experience, and the sociable role members provide counterbalancing positive support.

Stage 3 deals with introspective themes that are reflected in mechanisms involving greater autonomy. Because the work of this stage is less interpersonal in nature, role functions are less central. Sociable and divergent role members encourage the opening process, whereas structural and cautionary role members try to understand the internal material being revealed.

Stage 4 is concerned with intimacy issues, which are worked out between the positive orientation of the sociable and structural role members, and the negative tendencies of the divergent and cautionary role members.

Stage 5 represents a shift back to autonomy and responsibility. Here the alignments change, with the structural and cautionary role members promoting individual autonomy themes, and the sociable and divergent role members seeking greater interdependence.

Note how the principal axis between stage 1 and stage 2, as well as that between stages 4 and 5, shifts 90 degrees. This graphically demonstrates the idea that the second of each sequence, stages 2 and 5, respectively, addresses the tensions of the preceding stage by providing an alternative perspective on the importance of group events.

Termination is welcomed by the cautionary role members and most regretted by the sociable role members.

The connections between developmental stages and social roles can be illustrated with a map based on the idea of interpersonal dimensions. One such system that has come into recent use in psychotherapy research is the Structural Analysis of Social Behavior (SASB). The SASB system is a modified two-axial circumplex (circular) model of personality, a method of conceptualizing interpersonal functioning that has a long tradition. SASB is based on the idea of two bipolar dimensions of social interaction: affiliation/rejection and independence/interdependence (Figure 5-1). More detail concerning the SASB system is provided in Note 96.

This system is proving to be surprisingly versatile in capturing the complexity of human interactions. It will be used throughout this book as a map of interpersonal space on which to plot concepts such

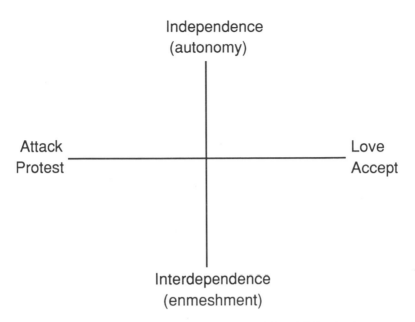

Figure 5-1. The two axes of Structural Analysis of Social Behavior interpersonal system.

as developmental stages, social roles, and critical incidents. The advantage of adding this standard vocabulary to the usual clinical repertoire is that clinicians tend to use idiosyncratic expressions for describing people and their behavior that may not have the same meaning for others. A formal system such as SASB provides counterbalance to that possibility. Because it is based on an interpersonal theory of social behavior, it is well suited for use in a group context.

With the SASB system, the sequence of stage tasks can be seen to encompass a comprehensive sampling of role activities. These connections are portrayed schematically in Figure 5-2. There will be many subtleties and unique variations in any given group, but the overall patterns are useful in plotting major dimensions of the group process. The social roles are located in each quadrant as shown. The interactional dimension "in focus" during each stage bisects the SASB space, forming an axis of tension involving the nearest social role representatives. For example, the sociable role members lead the action in stage 1, and their efforts are most resisted by members demonstrating cautionary role behaviors. In stage 4, the positively oriented structural and sociable role members are in tension with the negatively oriented cautionary and divergent role members. Used in

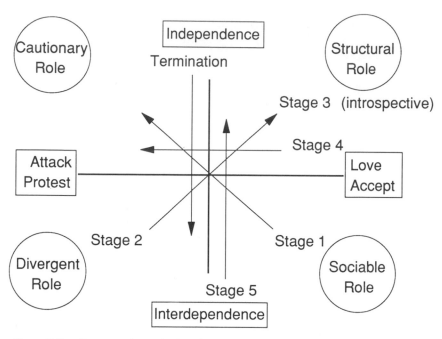

Figure 5-2.   Stages and social roles plotted in Structural Analysis of Social Behavior interactional space.

this way, the SASB space forms a framework for understanding the group and the relationship between the group and its members. The stage/role language may be used as a metaphor for conceptualizing broad themes and describing the group as a whole. Guidelines regarding behaviors to be reinforced or dampened are implicit in the descriptions of stages and roles. With this framework, the therapist is able to predict and react to group themes in a way that is likely to promote group development.

The material in Chapters 4 and 5 has dealt with group-level issues. The group therapist also needs to attend to the basic principles of individual psychotherapy. The outcome of group psychotherapy is not a successful group, but successfully changed individual members. The therapist must be prepared to shift between understanding group-level issues and understanding the individual. The group phenomena described in this section are characteristic of all groups. For psychotherapeutic work, these ideas must be integrated with considerations of the individual motivations underlying the behavior of each member.

The Early Group

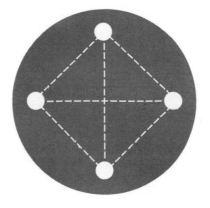

CHAPTER 6

Assessment

This chapter begins the process of applying the basic group theory of Section I to clinical work. The sequence of the topics in this chapter follows that actually used during the assessment process itself. First, assessment of prospective group members entails a consideration of formal diagnosis and relative contraindications. Then, the assessment must match the needs and capacity of the individual with the type of group to be formed. The final portion of the chapter is devoted to the more detailed assessment required for groups that will emphasize active psychological learning from the interactional experience among the group members, that is, for interpersonal or psychodynamic groups. Several techniques are described for establishing a focus for such therapeutic work.

Diagnostic Considerations

Formal Diagnosis

A formal diagnostic assessment should precede the decision to place a patient in a therapy group. This material is written with the assumption that the reader is able to make a careful diagnosis based on *Diagnostic and Statistical Manual of Mental Disorders, Third Edition, Revised* (DSM-III-R), Axis I criteria. There are many issues that go into the decision to place a patient in group psychotherapy, but a fundamental starting point is a firm diagnostic opinion. It might be argued that group therapy does not treat diagnoses, it treats people. And indeed this is true. However, the group therapist needs to be in a position to predict likely downside risks for a given patient, and diagnosis is a great help.

The assessment should identify conditions for which there are other specific treatments that may precede, accompany, or replace group psychotherapy. It should also detect specific contraindications to the use of group therapy. The group therapist should know if a potential group member is suffering from an organic impairment of thought processing; psychotic phenomena from an organic, schizophrenic, or affective condition; a major affective disorder; or phobic or panic symptoms. Specific treatments are indicated for these conditions. Group approaches may be still useful for many of these patients, but the diagnosis will affect the type of group and the choice of therapist strategy. These issues will be discussed further when we come to the matter of group composition.

The above major clusters of diagnoses do not include most of the anxiety-related disorders, which constitute a large percentage of outpatient referrals, nor do they include patients with dysthymic diagnoses. These are "upset" people who usually present with features of anxiety, unhappiness, and demoralization associated with low self-esteem. Such symptoms are usually embedded in situations of interpersonal distress.

Axis II personality features are open to much greater variability of clinical judgment. Later in this chapter, some interesting ways are reviewed to address the task of interpersonal functioning. The dimensions described are useful additions to the categories of Axis II. However, it is important to determine the depth of dysfunction associated with characterologic features. This is best evaluated not by symptoms but by general social adaptation, including a history of instability in work or education, a lack of reasonably satisfying involvement in social activities, legal or criminal problems, and multiple brief or chaotic close relationships (29).

Looking at assessment from a different perspective, several specific goals can be identified. In order of priority, these tasks include 1) to rule out group approaches for a given patient, 2) to decide on the type of group that would be most appropriate, 3) to make decisions about group composition, 4) to predict group behavior including assets or liabilities that are likely to be encountered, and 5) to consider therapeutic strategies that might be used. These matters are discussed in this chapter and the next.

Relative Contraindications for Group Therapy

Need for low-stimulation environment.   The first exclusion criteria to apply is whether the patient can tolerate an arousing environment. Sitting in a room with a number of people and the expectation of participation in a group is a reasonably high–stimulation environment. It is contraindicated for patients who are actively manic or extremely labile and for whom a low-stimulation environment is desirable. At some point when the patient begins to slow down, the opportunity to reflect on the manic episode in a group may be indicated. Clinical judgment is required for patients in a hypomanic state who may want to be in the ward group, but who begin to escalate once they are in it. The therapist should forewarn such patients that they may find the group a little much to handle initially and that they can leave, or be asked to leave, if that proves to be the case.

Inability to attend to process.   Patients in an acutely agitated state are unsuitable. They simply cannot be reasonably expected to benefit from what a group has to offer. This includes agitation related to organic factors such as major withdrawal symptoms, an acute schizophrenic presentation, or an acutely excited state due to stimulant substance abuse. This does not refer to the presence of psychotic symptoms per se, but rather to the ability to tolerate sitting in a room and attending at a basic level to what is going on.

Paranoid style.   A patient who characteristically uses intense projective defenses is unlikely to benefit from a group setting. The presence of a high degree of suspicion and an orientation of hypervigilance toward the environment precludes use of the interpersonal exchange modalities on which a group depends. The nature of the paranoid defense is to reflect, not absorb, personal comments. The paranoid individual therefore does not learn from the group interaction, only reacts against it. Groups may struggle for hours trying to penetrate such defenses. This can be demoralizing to the members and potentially damaging to the recipient. Such patients usually do not recognize their tendency to distort and may need to be tactfully directed into other treatment approaches. These comments refer to an enduring characterologic style. They do not apply to an acute reactive state in which paranoid defenses may be temporarily mobilized, nor to an acute paranoid psychotic episode. As such patients begin to recover, they may find a group quite helpful in guiding them through a process of reality testing.

Brittle denial.   Similarly, a patient who uses extremely brittle denial defenses may be unable to use group interaction constructively. As with projective defenses, denial blocks receptivity. On the other hand, group members are often more successful than an individual therapist in breaking through moderate levels of denial because there is less role status involved. Therefore, denial is not an absolute contraindication to group therapy, but rather something to be assessed on an individual basis.

Schizoid traits.   Severe character pathology in the schizoid range seriously interferes with the patient's ability to use a social therapy. Such patients by definition are not motivated to work toward interpersonal openness, and they actively avoid closeness. They tend to do poorly with any of the talking therapies. Fortunately, they seldom present for psychotherapeutic treatments unless brought by family or spouse. A history of very isolated adaptation with which the individual is quite content should be taken seriously. It is generally not difficult to separate such a history from that presented by an avoidant personality style, in which the person is fearful of relationships but wants to develop them.

Antisocial personality.   A well-documented diagnosis of antisocial personality disorder in an adult constitutes reasonable grounds for exclusion from a general therapy group. An exception to this is a specialized group primarily devoted to such characterologic problems. The decision to exclude such a person from a group may be hotly contested. Assessment of character pathology is not an absolute science, and such patients can be obliging and apparently accessible for psychological discussion. They may charm a group in the initial stages only to turn into a destructive force later. Fortunately, the diagnostic criteria for antisocial personality contained in DSM-III-R are reasonably effective in confirming a diagnosis. The major problem is differentiating an "acting out" reactive state from an enduring trait. Documentation of significant dysfunction extending back into adolescent years is helpful in this regard.

Primitive character pathology. Serious questions must also be raised about including patients with primitive characterologic styles falling in the borderline-narcissistic area in therapy groups. The interactional stimulation of a group will fan the flames of such psychopathology. The presence of a reactive audience may positively reinforce excessive emotional displays and interpersonal manipulation. The result is intensification of problems with impulse control and the appearance of gross distortions in interpersonal evaluations and social judgment. Splitting and projective identification mechanisms can be expected that may fragment the group or isolate the leader.

A fundamental decision in the management of such patients entails the choice between an intense psychotherapeutic approach and a supportive strategy of behavioral containment and dampening. These patients may benefit from brief inpatient care, but this effect is primarily related to the "time-out" features of hospitalization, perhaps enhanced with low doses of neuroleptic medication. This rationale is reinforced by keeping their involvement in the ward milieu to a minimum without participation in ward groups. These views may seem somewhat heretical in this heyday of enthusiasm for borderline phenomena. However, there is minimal evidence that shorter-term approaches of a psychotherapeutic nature make a significant impact on the patient, and they often lead to major problems for the other group members.

These cautionary remarks are not meant to apply to specialized settings where specific programs are designed with borderline patients in mind. But these are predicated on longer-term interventions and sophisticated staff who are able to deal constructively with the management issues posed. In such a context, group therapy is not only indicated but may be the most powerful component of the experience. However, such group applications require advanced therapy skills and are beyond the scope of an introductory text.

The evaluation of character pathology is made more difficult because patients are usually assessed at a point of relative decompensation when characterologic style is exaggerated. They have become caricatures of their usual selves. A careful longitudinal history and efforts to find third-party confirmation of historical information are invaluable for comparing present state with usual adaptation levels.

Demographic Variables

There are consistent correlations between social class and premature termination from therapy. Patients in social class 5, the lowest, have a particularly high dropout rate. On the other hand, if such patients remain in treatment, their outcome is equal to that of higher social classes. These findings suggest the need for specific strategies to prepare patients in lower socioeconomic classes for therapy. The first few sessions are the time of highest risk for premature termination. In the next chapter, a model for pretherapy preparation is discussed. This is particularly important when social class or cultural issues may work against the idea of group psychotherapy.

Age and gender do not appear to be significant predictors of psychotherapy outcome. Although some of the older literature suggests that intelligence is an important selection criteria, experience suggests that, with the exception of clear subnormality, it has minimal predictive value. Of course, all of these demographic variables may be useful to consider in regard to group composition.

Types of Groups

Once a decision has been made that the patient is suitable for group psychotherapy, the next task is to decide what type of group is indicated. Inpatient groups will use relatively insensitive criteria, mainly the exclusion criteria above. Long-term dynamic psychotherapy groups in which personal responsibility for introspective and interpersonal work is expected will use criteria of finer sensitivity. Between these two extremes is a large gray area that will have to be decided on the merits of any given situation. This will involve some compromise between individual need, therapist skill, and availability of potential group members. Without pretending to be absolute about the divisions, the following types of groups might form a starting point for consideration.

Social skills. These groups are designed for patients with gross deficiency in basic social skills, often in the context of long-term psychiatric morbidity. An active and controlling leadership role is appropriate, and limited interactional behavior is expected of the members. Such groups make high use of the "supportive" cluster of therapeutic factors, often requiring the leader to repeatedly model these. Specific homework tasks are assigned, which are graded to each member's capabilities. Full use may be made of extending the group atmosphere into the community through planned activities among the members between sessions. These groups are often found in conjunction with a broader range of rehabilitation approaches such as supervised accommodation and sheltered workshops.

Cognitive focus.   This includes groups with a high educational component, such as post–heart–attack programs. Cognitive-behavioral techniques are often applied in a group setting, for example with depressed patients. Behavioral management of anxiety or phobic problems by means of relaxation techniques and life-style planning discussions can be helpful. In these groups, full use is made of the supportive cluster of therapeutic factors. Active interaction appropriate to stage 1 is an important ingredient, and the therapist may actively intervene to keep the group at this level. These groups often have a larger membership and are leader oriented.

Interpersonal—restitutive.   Active interpersonal work is expected, and the goal is to master a current stress, for example the loss of a spouse or adjustment to college. The focus is on mastery of the situation, not on personal change. It may happen that successful management of a difficult situation will set in motion important enduring changes, but this is not the principal goal of the group. These groups are often of a brief nature and may serve as a prelude to referral for more intensive therapy.

Interpersonal—explorative.   The expected focus is on recurrent interpersonal patterns that interfere with satisfactory intimate relationships. Active introspective work is expected, and it is anticipated that the experience will raise anxiety, not dampen it. The interactions among the group members will be a major area for therapeutic activity. Groups with these goals vary considerably in duration. Historically, they have tended to be longer term, perhaps 1 or 2 years or more. Often such groups are of a slow-open nature, with members being added from time to time but the actual group running indefinitely. More recently, there have been reports of much briefer groups of 12–20 sessions in which intensive interpersonal work is expected. These brief groups are usually closed, with all members beginning and ending together.

It is immediately clear that there will be considerable overlap between these categories and that no neatly distinguishing lines can be drawn. However, this list does form a hierarchy of expectations regarding the psychological depth of personal work and the extent to which interpersonal learning will be applied. As one goes down the list, the degree of anxiety stimulated by the experience increases. These levels provide some guidelines for placing members with similar expectations together, resulting in greater group cohesion and more effective use of group interaction.

Personal Dimensions

Diagnostic categories begin to lose their usefulness as one moves down the above list of levels of group work. More subtle aspects of psychological functioning become more pertinent. These characteristics will help in the process of setting realistic goals, choosing the most appropriate type of group, and making group composition decisions. They are similar to the assessment dimensions used for individual psychotherapy (30).

Capacity to Relate

Assessment of the capacity to relate is based on evidence that the patient is able to engage in meaningful relationships, that is, ones in which the patient experiences elements of trust, responsibility, and altruistic give-and-take. A history of important relationships extending over periods of time is sought. Even though these may eventually have an unsatisfactory ending, the ability to form them is the operative criterion. Historical information concerning the family of origin is useful to elicit, particularly the presence of an enduring nurturing figure. However, such information is subject to considerable distortion in the reporting.

Harder data are found through careful observation of the patient's behavior in the assessment interview. The interviewer may look for the patient's capacity to speak openly about interpersonal issues, to allow the interviewer some degree of emotional closeness, to react collaboratively and flexibly to the demands of the assessment task, and to experience and express affect in the interview. These qualities suggest an ability to establish a relationship that contains a degree of basic trust and confidence in the ultimate benevolence and helpfulness of the therapist.

Such an assessment is likely to identify those patients who are markedly schizoid or paranoid. It will also detect patients who are extremely defensive or who use brittle levels of denial. Bear in mind the adage, "One doesn't build iron cages for mice." To some extent, the assessment process is appropriately based on a "feel" of connectedness with the patient that is difficult to fully describe. When the interviewer comes out of an assessment interview with the feeling that there has been no meaningful contact with the other person, that hunch should be carefully taken into account.

Psychological Mindedness

Psychological mindedness may be rated on a spectrum. This begins with the ability to simply label internal states: "I recognize that I am unhappy." Some patients, for example those with many somatic symptoms, may have difficulty even at this stage. They may be said to suffer from "alexithymia"—no words for describing emotion. The next step in psychological mindedness is an appreciation that emotional states may be related to needs or wishes: "I am unhappy because I am lonely." At the next level, causal links can be made: "I get headaches every time I visit my mother." Recognition of hidden motivations or mixed feelings represents further sophistication: "Sometimes I can't stand my father, and other times I really need to go home."

Being able to connect such "conflicted" states with an underlying fear or anxiety represents greater psychological mindedness. Higher levels are reflected in an appreciation that tension or anxiety may be motivating behavior, not just signaling a response to difficult situations. Recognition of defensive maneuvers of a self-protecting nature to avoid addressing the conflictual focus is more advanced. The ability to relate such ideas to past experiences and to the assessment interview itself offers even stronger evidence for suitability. Such qualities help to establish a working focus for the therapy, particularly when the patient can acknowledge therapeutic goals in terms of personal psychological change.

Patients with higher levels of psychological mindedness are more likely to complete brief group psychotherapy. This does not necessarily imply that patients with lower psychological mindedness should not enter group therapy, but rather that their acceptance into groups in which interpersonal insightful work is expected needs to be carefully considered. They may need extra preparation to enhance their ability to use the work of the group to best advantage (31).

At the time of assessment, high levels of insight are not expected, but rather a general ability to consider psychological issues. The therapist should carefully probe the patient's expectations about how treatment might help. A serious misalignment with regard to the importance of personal psychological factors will sabotage the progress of therapy, in terms of both the likelihood of engagement in the group process and the ability to focus on specific target areas. For example, a patient may anticipate that the group experience will be like a social club in which friends will be made and entertainment planned, or a patient may expect to receive only medication and support.

Trial interpretations.   These are designed to test the patient's response to psychologically minded ideas. This provides first-hand information about the likelihood of engagement in necessary therapeutic tasks. Is the patient able to take an interpretation and work with it, or does it lead to heightened defensiveness and a drop in rapport?

Trial interpretations include statements in which the interviewer links the patient's behavior with possible internal motivations: "It sounds as if you really wanted to be taken care of but got angry instead." The interviewer may make connections between stressful events and the onset of symptoms: "Do I hear you saying that each time you phoned him you got a headache?" Parallels may be drawn between recurring maladaptive patterns and relationships that occur over time: "This recent relationship seems to have ended the same way several others did." Some aspects of the interview process itself may be reflected: "I wondered what it was like for you when I kept coming back to that difficult period."

Such interpretations should be presented in a tentative and exploratory fashion, as an attempt to encourage the patient to clarify the issues, not as a confrontation that can be rejected. They are an opportunity to see if the patient is able to become a collaborating ally in the exploration process, not an attempt to create instant insight. They will also provide information about the patient's ability to focus on specific interpersonal issues, rather than viewing the situation in vague and general terms. It is best if they are directed at a level that is close to the patient's level of understanding.

Motivation

The term *motivation* should be used in reference to the patient's willingness, not capacity, to participate in the tasks of therapy. In particular, the patient should express some interest in participating in a group. Most patients view the idea of group therapy with considerable apprehension. Some have an absolute block about the matter that may be difficult to overcome. Most are willing to give it a try, especially if the clinician shows no hesitation about the recommendation. But the question of group therapy needs to be specifically addressed in the assessment process. In a general sense, the patient should be willing to look inward (introspect), to be willing to try out new ways of relating, and to acknowledge that trying to understand behavior might be of value. These aspects of motivation are directly connected to the process of alignment regarding the tasks of therapy.

Some patients have great difficulty in tolerating the idea of sitting in a group and have a fear of "group contagion," which may mount to phobic levels. Although such reactions usually settle eventually, the initial reaction may be such as to preclude involvement in the group. If coerced into a group, the result may be rapid termination with highly negative views of the process.

The patient must also be willing to make sacrifices in terms of time, effort, and money to attend therapy sessions regularly. The projected duration of therapy and the frequency and duration of sessions all need to be carefully laid out and the patient's agreement to full participation obtained. This is often couched in terms of expecting a commitment to attend so many sessions, often 12, before making any decisions about dropping out. This is best put in terms of a trial period before considering a decision to drop out, not an initial period after which the contract is renewed. This avoids providing an inviting opportunity for patients to use the commitment concept as a rationale for discontinuing therapy.

A careful review of the process by which the patient arrived for assessment may reveal that the true source of motivation lies elsewhere, perhaps in the spouse, parent, or employer. If important motivational or influencing factors involve the family, then an assessment at that level needs to be made. When an intact family system is available, care should be taken not to ignore factors within it that sustain the pathological adaptation or that may be useful in addressing it. The group system is a powerful force for change. However, the patient's real social system should always be given priority because it operates 24 hours a day, 7 days a week. Therapy for the individual may be useful, but the odds of it having a beneficial effect can be increased when the outside system is also working in a constructive direction.

Adaptational Strengths

During the assessment process, the general level of the patient's adaptation during successive life stages should be surveyed. This is based on the not unreasonable assumption that consistency in education and work, social stability, and the absence of periods of severe psychological decompensation all provide evidence of a general ability to adapt to life's vicissitudes. A history of general stability, even in the face of poor intimate relationships, makes it more likely that the patient will tolerate the early stages of therapy and thus have access to the effects of group therapeutic factors.

Attention must also be given to the identification of positive personality assets. Because time-limited psychotherapy deals with a limited range of problems, it is particularly important that the patient's strengths be selectively reinforced. The interviewer can identify such strengths through the assessment of effective problem-solving skills, determination and persistence in addressing problems, and evidence of effective mediation between internal pressures and external realities in some, if not all, areas of functioning. It is useful for the therapist to carefully keep these positive issues in mind so that they can be used within the group for motivational and support functions.

Other Treatment Experiences

Information about what has helped the patient on other occasions is very helpful. If the patient has been in four previous groups and dropped out of each after a few sessions, the data need to be weighed seriously. The odds will be stacked against even the world's most charismatic therapist. A history of rapid response to antidepressants with satisfying personal relationships between episodes might encourage a focus on biological, not psychotherapeutic, interventions. The response to past treatment may provide useful ideas about how the patient understands improvement to occur. It also may reveal some quite specific information. For example, it may emerge that the patient is currently being treated elsewhere and has sought consultation because that therapy was beginning to focus on difficult issues.

As a general rule, patients involved in a current major life stressor, such as divorce or recent bereavement, are best not placed in a group in which intensive interpersonal learning is anticipated. Realistic preoccupation with the external event will interfere with an introspective process. It will also elicit the sympathy of other members, making productive confrontation less likely. Groups of a supportive nature may be helpful. It is useful to bear in mind that most people successfully cope with life's adversities. Therapy groups are indicated for those who become blocked in the working-through process.

The final issue that must be assessed from the history is the risk of severe decompensation. What is the worst the patient has ever been and what were the circumstances? Is it likely that the patient when stressed in a group may decompensate into an actively suicidal state? Is there a past history of such incidents following interpersonal difficulties? Such developments will not only preoccupy much of the group's time, but may actually frighten other members from tackling important issues. Does the patient have a past history of poor impulse control with destructive or self-destructive behavior when confronted with a frustrating situation? Such events may leave other group members feeling guilty or ambivalently angry. Alcohol or substance abuse may result in a patient showing up for therapy in a state that precludes effective utilization of group sessions.

Establishing an Interpersonal Focus

Interpersonal phenomena form the basic infrastructure of group psychotherapy. One of the tasks for the group therapist is to move between an intrapsychic individual perspective and an interpersonal transactional language. A central therapeutic strategy is to maximize learning from the here-and-now group events. The stage for this can be set during the assessment process by emphasizing psychological goals for the individual in terms of interpersonal issues. This does not deny the realm of internal mechanisms but chooses to look at the results of these as enacted in relationships. An interpersonal focus is defined as a recurrent interpersonal theme underlying dysfunctional relationships. This theme, once identified, becomes the central focus for therapeutic work. It both limits and concentrates the field of action. This is particularly important in time-limited approaches because the time frame allows less opportunity for corrective realignment during the course of therapy.

Interpersonal Measures

Many of the following ideas are drawn from the individual psychotherapy research literature. This work is of particular interest because, in the service of better interrater reliability, most investigators have come to use interpersonal measures. These research projects have a strong grounding in clinical work, and their techniques serve to sharpen perception and encourage focusing on critical dimensions. The clinician can use some of these ideas not in a stringent research protocol fashion, but to augment clinical judgment. The five interpersonal measures discussed below seem particularly well adapted for use with group psychotherapy.

Core Conflictual Relationship Theme (CCRT). This method, developed by Luborsky in the Penn psychotherapy project, tries to capture the essence of a relationship by fitting it to a standard format:

> I (the patient) wish/need/intend _____
> from _____ (the other), BUT _____.

The first part of the statement is the core theme of the relationship. The *but* represents an attempted solution to the achievement of the interpersonal wish. This solution may or may not be adaptive. Answers to the *but* may be subdivided into answers that focus on the response of others, such as, "But he will reject me if I express my affection," and those that focus on the response of the self, such as, "But I may lose control if I begin to show my anger."

To arrive at a valid CCRT statement, it is necessary to sample 8–10 relationships. A 1-hour therapy session usually offers pretty close to this number of relationship episodes. Each of these consists of an interpersonal vignette, a "short story" in which the patient describes a relationship with another. To develop the CCRT presented below, a simple semistructured interview was used. The patient was asked to describe some actual event between himself and each of eight important people in his life, including each parent. Each vignette was then scored using the "I wish BUT . . ." format. In seven of the eight stories, the same theme emerged.

This procedure is really only a slightly formalized way of taking a personal life history. Assessments routinely contain information of this nature in a less structured format. In fact, after having become familiar with this technique, history taking becomes more fun as one searches for the elusive *but*. This entails placing emphasis on the meaning of the events or the relationship that is being described: "What did it mean to you when he left abruptly like that?" "What do you think she thought of you after you said that?" This sounds like good sensitive interviewing, doesn't it?

A brief case history is described in Table 6-1, along with a CCRT formulation that summarizes the responses on the eight vignettes. This case will be used later in the book to demonstrate the relationship between assessment findings and therapeutic tasks.

The CCRT shown in Table 6-1 suggests a systematic intrusive trend toward seeing relationships in dangerous terms and therefore the need for help and protection. This is associated with a self-critical attitude and attempts to solve the need by avoiding involvement with people.

Luborsky has found that patients consistently repeat the core theme across various relationships, just as authors work on a common theme across a lifetime of novels. The core theme does not change as the result of therapy; however, changes occur in the *but* solution to the thematic wish. Patients with positive outcomes show not only a reduction in symptoms but a significant shift from negative to positive solutions, and the solutions represent a more effective problem-solving style (32).

Configurational analysis.   Horowitz uses an approach that is in some ways similar to Luborsky's CCRT. In studying videotapes of therapy sessions, he noted how patients could click into different relationship modes, a phenomenon he called "states of mind." Each state reflects an interactional tendency that can be described in terms of overt behavior, emotional qualities, level of control, and defensive arrangements. Issues related to self-concept, role relationship models, and conflictual relationship schemes can be added to the description of each state. Once a series of states has been identified for an individual, attention is focused on the triggering events that appear to promote a change from one state to another, including the effect of therapist interventions. This expands the field from Luborsky's single core theme to a handful of characteristic states. Different therapeutic strategies may be described for each state, and typical states may be found in particular personality configurations (33).

For example, the man whose CCRT was described in Table 6-1 could be described in terms of the role-relationship model that he applied to his relationships with women. He found himself involved in a series of intimate relationships with women whom he perceived as controlling. He would react to this by intermittently, and inappropriately, having to demonstrate his ability to decide situations. When this was not possible, he would shift into a nonchalant uncaring state in which he avoided all semblance of involvement.

Table 6-1.   Case history with subsequent Core Conflictual Relationship Theme
(CCRT)

Case History

The patient is a 38-year-old single man with an advanced university degree who works as a successful self-employed artist. He presented with a depressed mood, stating that he did not know where his life was going and he could not get organized to do anything productive. He described fluctuating depressions since his early 20s, usually triggered by relationship stresses. He denied any suicidal ideation at the time of assessment, but later admitted that he had come very close to a lethal suicide attempt.

He described his mother as a caring but ineffectual woman, and his father as aloof and nonsupportive. He recognized that as a child he wanted their approval, yet chronically underachieved. He gave a history of four significant relationships with women, including a current one, in which he felt too controlled.

He had therapy briefly during graduate school in response to the termination of his first serious relationship. He had been seen elsewhere in supportive therapy for several months before this assessment. It emerged that the present referral was for a consideration of medication. It was felt that he did not have a major affective disorder and that the referral reflected termination control issues with the previous therapist.

CCRT Formulation

WISH: I need to be helped, protected, and comforted.

Response of others—Negative:
    They are violent toward me.
    They get angry at me.
    They are frustrated with me.
Response of others—Positive:
    They protect me.
    They comfort me.
    They save my life.
    They are united in their concern over me.
Response of self—Negative:
    I am fearful for my personal safety.
    I fear for the death of others.
Response of self—Positive:
    I feel secure.
    I am different.
Response of self—Unexpressed:
    I am stupid and inadequate.
    I do not live up to others' expectations.
    I will not ask for help.

Interpersonal content themes. Klerman has described a model developed for the treatment of depressed patients. Relationship themes are extracted from diagnostic summaries. A person may be placed in one of four categories based on thematic content: grief, interpersonal disputes, role transitions, and interpersonal deficits. Each category is linked to specific intervention strategies. Although these categories originated in a research approach restricted to depression, it is clear that the categories themselves may be applied in a broad range of psychotherapeutic situations in which issues of loss, disappointment, fear, and demoralization are found (34).

The patient in Table 6-1 falls into the category of interpersonal disputes. At first glance, the history of recurrent depressions in association with failing relationships might lead one to postulate the category of grief. However, a careful review of the sequence of events indicates that interpersonal issues arose first, and only when the relationship reached an impasse did the reactive depressed state emerge.

Life-stage developmental issues. Another way for defining an interpersonal focus is with the language of adult development. One advantage of this perspective is that it promotes a basically positive orientation to therapy. The role of the therapist is seen as helping to remove blocks that stand in the way of natural maturational processes. Therapy gives a boost to powerful developmental forces. This perspective implies that once a small shift has occurred, the working-through process will proceed under its own momentum without the need for extensive ongoing therapy. This view is very much in harmony with systems theory. Budman has advocated incorporating this attitude into the process of group composition. By putting people together who are dealing with similar developmental issues, he is able to mobilize strong cohesive forces (35).

From this perspective, our patient is dealing with relatively advanced issues. He has demonstrated his capacity to establish intimate adult relationships, but finds himself in difficulty regarding dominance and control issues, which then sabotage the union.

Structural Analysis of Social Behavior (SASB). The measurement of personality and interpersonal behavior is a controversial area, one in which there is a diversity of strongly held opinions. The SASB system was introduced in Chapter 5 as a device for organizing the ideas of stages and roles in terms of interpersonal dimensions. When the vignettes of the patient presented in Table 6-1 are scored with SASB, they suggest an underlying theme of feared attack to which the patient reacts with either a desperate search for a protecting figure or an overdetermined need to control. When this does not work, his recourse is to move into a position of distancing and isolation. In some circumstances, critical comments from others are converted into strong self-blaming ideas. Figure 6-1 demonstrates these patterns as they emerged in the transcripts of his vignettes regarding significant relationships.

These five perspectives offer various ways to develop an interpersonal focus. Of course, the well-established practice of making a dynamic formulation has the same goal. The value of thinking through some of these more structured techniques is that they can sharpen clinical focus and draw attention to matters that might otherwise be missed.

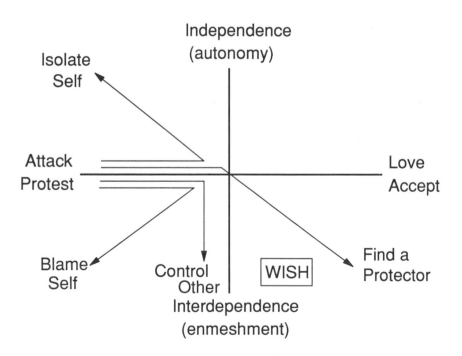

Figure 6-1. Structural Analysis of Social Behavior used to analyze content of vignettes in case history found in Table 6-1.

Negotiating an Interpersonal Focus

No matter what systematic or inferential process is used to define the therapeutic focus in clinical practice, it is important that it be based on a process of open dialogue. The interviewer may guide the discussion toward what appear to be relevant issues, but the final decision must be mutual. One result of the assessment procedure should be a clearly stated contract with the patient about the principal focus. During therapy, the patient may be expected to make attempts to ignore or circumvent this focus, and an agreement established at the beginning is useful in dealing with such events. Therapy is more effective when attention is consistently paid to the focal issue. We shall consider how to use this assessment work to greatest advantage in the following chapters.

The assessment process is the first experience the patient has with the therapeutic environment. The sorts of issues that are of interest to the interviewer will signal the direction in which therapy is expected to go. Thus, in a very real sense, the assessment process is the beginning of therapy. It also prepares the patient for the types of interactions that are going to be of greatest value during the therapy. By concentrating on interpersonal meaning in a personal historical sense and in terms of group process, the therapist and the members are driven to deal openly with the here-and-now experiences of the group.

This chapter has been written from the standpoint of assessment being conducted by the future group leader. This is not always the case. When assessments are done by a different clinician, the categories of information discussed in this chapter should be systematically reported. The attitude of the person doing the assessment is also important. The process should still be considered to be part of pretherapy preparation, and the relevance of the material elicited to the group work should be emphasized. This can be accomplished by statements such as, "Your group therapist will be particularly interested in . . . ," or "You will find in the group that your ability to put your thoughts into words will be very useful." Even if the assessment for group referral is made by an independent clinician, a strong argument can be made for some individual contact, however brief, with the group therapist before a patient enters a group.

Summary

A careful assessment is a prerequisite to beginning group therapy. This should include a formal diagnostic opinion and a screening for contraindications to group involvement. One major purpose of an assessment is to determine what type of group would be most important. Patients being considered for groups in which active interpersonal work is expected require more extensive assessment. This includes several additional measures of suitability as well as an effort to determine a focus for therapeutic work. Structured assessment approaches are available that may be of value to the clinician.

CHAPTER 7

Composition and Preparation

This chapter moves from the level of the individual patient to a consideration of group composition. This shifts the discussion up one level in the organizational hierarchy, moving from the individual to conceptualize clinical decisions in terms of group-level issues. A pretherapy preparation format is introduced as well as specific planning for the first session. Careful attention to these preliminary details will be rewarded by the rapid development of a cohesive group.

Criteria for Composition

Composition—Homogeneity

There are diverse opinions concerning the principles of group composition (36). Some claim to take all comers, whereas others try for quite specific homogeneity in choosing members. It is likely that almost all groups are composed with some idea of homogeneity in mind. This may not be made explicit because some service settings automatically impose constraints on the sorts of people likely to become members. For example, groups formed in college health service programs are likely to have considerable homogeneity in terms of the central themes to be addressed. Groups on locked wards of state hospitals will have many patients with common diagnoses. In short, in the real world, homogeneity will be hard to avoid. Nonetheless, in fact because of these built-in possibilities, the basis of homogeneity should be examined for its suitability. For example, on a substance abuse unit, there may be several unique subpopulations residing under that general diagnostic umbrella.

This book is primarily oriented toward time-limited groups. With this approach, it is particularly useful to think of composing groups according to some principle of homogeneity. When the group is set up so that the members have some common issues, the engagement process can move faster. It is easier for members to begin interacting because they can knowledgeably share similar concerns and can become involved with each other on the basis of common experiences. Thus the group can master stage 1 tasks in a shorter time period.

The advantages of homogeneity extend beyond early group interaction. If members have experienced similar stressful events or similar dysfunctional behaviors, they are in a good position to recognize themselves in others. They are able to identify methods of resistance or label mixed messages more easily. They cannot fall back on the rationale that "you can't understand me because you haven't experienced what I have." Indeed, the opposite is the case, issues can be understood only too well. Therefore, for time-limited groups, there is a strong recommendation that some aspect of homogeneity be incorporated into composition decisions. There are a number of issues that may be considered as a basis for homogeneity.

Therapeutic goals.   The first issue to be considered with some care is what the goals of the group are to be. In Chapter 6, it was suggested that assessment be made in terms of suitability for levels of expected group process: social skills, cognitive tasks, mastery of a current stressful situation, or interpersonal exploratory work. These four levels constitute one way of defining a homogeneous component for composition. They constitute a continuum in regard to the use of intrusive interaction among the members. As one moves along this continuum, the requirement for greater selectivity goes up. If the group is going to have a largely educative format, then composition issues are of minimal importance apart from the material being of relevance to the members. A group that hopes to move into vigorous psychotherapeutic work will need more careful selection. The first concern in thinking of group composition is to review realistically what the objectives of the group experience should be. These are best committed to paper, which ensures that the issues are clarified and can be applied systematically to each potential member.

Diagnostic category.   Group composition is frequently based on diagnostic homogeneity. There is almost no limit to examples. The
most common theme in outpatient groups is concern about problems
of getting comfortably close to people or of being able to be one's own
person in a relationship. There are some advantages to treating patients with eating disorders in homogeneous groups. Other groups
have been composed of people having difficulty in adjusting to a
recent loss. Groups for substance abusers have a long history and are
often tailored to the characteristics of specific chemical agents, such
as alcohol, cocaine, or tranquilizer medications, and their users. Inpatient groups may be based on the members having in common the
experience of psychotic phenomena such as hallucinations or delusions. Behaviorally oriented therapists use groups for providing relaxation or desensitizing protocols for patients with phobias. Many
groups have been successful in helping patients cope with the adjustment to physical illness, for example, the unique stresses of long-term
renal dialysis or extensive burns, or the multisystem effects of dia-
betes mellitus. This list could go on indefinitely as a testimony to the
importance of homogeneity based on diagnosis. Each type of group
may have a characteristic atmosphere that reflects the types of people drawn to it.

Adult developmental stage.   Another approach to homogeneity is to
compose groups of patients dealing with similar developmental issues. Age defines different sets of life tasks that automatically incorporate relevant themes. In composing any group, developmental issues should be taken into account as one determinant of homogeneity
(37). Young people are commonly divided into separate groups for
preadolescent children, young adolescents, and adolescents over age
15. Young adults dealing with issues of separation from family of
origin and the need to establish adult intimate relationships form the
next developmental category. Patients in the 25–40 age range often
are dealing with recurrent failures in relationships or marital breakdown. Some are facing disillusionment with the accomplishment of
the ambitions of their youth. The age range of 40–60 brings its own
developmental challenges. Children are leaving home, marriages must
be renegotiated, and work stresses may be increasing. Groups for
patients over age 60 deal with issues of declining health, evaluation of
life accomplishments, loss of partners or friends, and questions of
one's own impending death.

Composition—Interactional Variety

After establishing a source of homogeneity, the therapist may then address the second major composition issue—interactional variety. The prediction of how a particular person will behave in group is not a highly developed science. Indeed, it is not uncommon to be surprised at how much a patient may change in the transition from individual office to group room. This is in part a tribute to the influence of context on behavior. Nonetheless, some efforts to achieve a balance of interactional types within a group are indicated. This builds into the group structure the likelihood of differences that will stimulate group work.

It is usually possible to make an educated guess after an assessment interview as to the patient's preferred style within intimate relationships. The Structural Analysis of Social Behavior (SASB) interpersonal space may be used as a way of organizing typical behaviors. One useful approach is to strive to compose a group that has within the collective membership some representation from each quadrant. From a group system perspective, this would mean that the group has within it the resources to enact each social role. Sometimes, conflictual issues can be plotted that highlight opposite ends of a dimension. For example, a college student who makes nightly calls home, yet when at home gets into endless rows with parents over the right to stay out late, is dealing with issues along the vertical independence/interdependence axis of the SASB model. With tongue in cheek, I claim to always compose my groups of three sociable role members, three structural role members, two divergent role members, and one cautionary role member. This stacks the group in favor of positive sustaining members while having the capability within the group of the stimulus provided by divergent members and the outside perspective of the reluctant cautionary members. Needless to say the "ideal group" is seldom found. Perhaps putting the equation the other way is more realistic. Try to have within the group at least two or three members who represent forces for cohesion and work.

Composition—The "Noah's Ark" Principle

The final stage of group composition consists of applying the "Noah's Ark" principle. Scan the proposed composition for members who stand out from the rest according to some characteristic. One pensioner in a group of young people. The only man in a group of eight women. The only black in a group of whites. The only unskilled laborer in a group of college-educated patients. The only one with a schizophrenic diagnosis in a group of neurotic patients. Every potential isolate needs to have someone with whom to identify. This need not necessarily be on the specific dimension of difference. The intent is to ensure that there are some viable links available. If these concerns cannot be addressed, then consideration should be given to deferring that person to another group in which some compatibility could be expected. On the other hand, these criteria must be applied with clinical judgment. It is impossible to fine-tune the membership on all accounts, and people often show surprising flexibility. The therapist has to estimate the degree of isolation that might be expected. Such a process of reflection, if it does not result in dropping the supposed isolate, at least will forewarn the therapist to monitor such developments closely in the early sessions of the group. The therapist can then be prepared to engineer universality experiences to the best extent possible.

There is another technical advantage to the Noah's Ark approach. An individual who often experiences a sense of isolation in social settings may use this for defensive purposes. By pairing that person with another who is dealing with similar issues, the opportunity is provided to address other matters of dysfunction. For example, a histrionic homosexual patient cannot use the argument, "You don't understand me because I'm gay," if there are one or two other homosexuals in the group who can address the general interpersonal features as matters independent of sexual orientation.

Size and Timing

The optimum size of the group will vary according to the goals. For groups directed at improving social skills or groups with a strong educational component, the membership may increase to up to 15 or even 20 members. This size allows the opportunity for questions and discussion but precludes a major focus on learning from interpersonal events. Such groups will of necessity be quite leader oriented. For groups that are designed for interpersonal learning, the size is best kept below 10 members. Many therapists will try to start a group with 8 or 9 members in the anticipation that 1 or 2 may not stay beyond the first few sessions. The group then will be at 6 or 7 members and can continue without the addition of more. It is not recommended to begin a group with a small number in the expectation that more members will be added gradually as they become available. This condemns the group to a continual reworking of engagement issues, a process that will have a major effect on group morale and commitment.

If the duration of the group is to be quite brief, e.g., 12 sessions, then it is best that new members not be added during its course. For longer time-limited groups, some accommodation must be made between the ideal of a closed group and the requirements of a service system. The entry of new members is always a critical time for a group. Some regression in level of functioning is inevitable, and the new members are at risk for being scapegoated. The management of open groups is discussed further in Chapter 14. Groups that are being run in an intensive program such as a day hospital may manage the regular addition of members more easily. A well-established milieu acts as a buffer and sustains both the group and the new members through the entry process. Even in this sort of atmosphere, there is something to be said for limiting the entry of new members to specific times, perhaps a weekly admission point.

Pretherapy Preparation

Having composed the group, the next task is to prepare the members for the beginning of the group. Pretherapy preparation results in fewer early dropouts and faster development of cohesion. The main purpose is to influence the development of stage 1 phenomena. After the first six to eight sessions, the effects of preparation are washed out by the actual experiences within the group. Preparation has two technical effects. It increases the likelihood that members will stay in the group long enough to have an exposure to therapeutic factors, mainly from the "supportive" cluster. Second, it assists in the development of therapeutic group norms. Often patterns that arise in the first few sessions come to establish the group's image and are difficult to change. This *primacy effect* phenomenon is well recognized in the social psychology literature. Once a behavior is in place, it takes far more effort to change it than was necessary to prompt it in the beginning. Some form of systematic orientation should be considered a necessary part of professional group practice (38).

The purpose of this preparation is to educate patients about what to expect in the group and how to get the most out of it. This provides them with some cognitive predictability, which is a major source of strength as the group begins to form. It helps to build a common set of attitudes and expectations, described as *role induction*, for how to be a successful group member. The major choice is between doing pretherapy preparation in a group setting or with individual patients. There are advantages to both. No matter which is used, patients will be anxious about joining a group, so it is important to repeat, repeat, repeat, the information.

Preparation in a Group

Pretherapy material can be presented to a group in several ways. The choice is partly dependent on service characteristics. Programs with large volumes of patients may have regular pretherapy preparation meetings. Sometimes the material is covered with the incoming members of a particular group. Some recommend doing this with a slightly larger number than will actually be in the group and using the pretherapy experience to make final decisions about group composition. Sometimes pretherapy sessions may include the members of more than one group.

The advantage of a group approach is that it makes the material to be covered more real. A structured series of group exercises permits a controlled entry into experiencing the group process, at the same time using that process as an educational tool. Such sessions may consist of a brief introduction about the history and theory of group psychotherapy and an opportunity for questions. Often this is followed by a series of structured group exercises. For example, members can talk in pairs for 5 minutes and then introduce each other to the group. This begins a process of self-disclosure as well as a level of group participation that is controlled and safe. A useful second exercise is to ask members to identify something they would like to change or understand better in their personal relationships. This begins to focus on central themes as a target for therapeutic work. Within the course of a pretherapy session, the material outlined in the Appendix can be systematically covered. Most programs use a single session for the purpose, perhaps allowing 2 hours. Some use two sessions, but anything more runs into the problem that the therapeutic process will have begun before the "official" group starts.

For the patient, it is the experiential component, the "getting one's toes wet" experience, that is the strongest recommendation for a group approach. It provides desensitization to a group environment, which helps to control early session anxiety and promotes the commitment to begin the therapy group. For the therapist, a group preparation session provides an opportunity to see the patient functioning within a group setting and the opportunity to make final decisions about group composition. A patient who clearly does not fit may be identified as unsuitable for a particular group. A patient who poses major problems with disruptions and does not respond to guidance may be deemed not yet ready for a group experience.

The clinician conducting the pretherapy group needs to be alert to identifying potential dropouts. Sometimes misunderstandings can arise and, if not addressed, may lead patients to resolve that they could never be in a group with a particular person. Such decisions may also reflect a resistance to wanting to look at issues raised during the session. These meetings may be considered "pretherapy" in nature, but for the patients it is the beginning of the group treatment process, and they may be frightened off at the idea of serious work. If there are any indications of such reactions, the leader must address them openly and quickly. If successful, this is a good education in dealing with process issues. If the patient decides to leave anyway, this was probably inevitable and perhaps better that it happen before the group formally begins.

Preparation of the Individual

There are also advantages for the group therapist to have a few meetings with each patient individually before beginning the group. This provides an opportunity for the development of the beginning of a therapeutic alliance, which can be an important sustaining factor for the patient during the early sessions. The danger is that the patient may then be resistant to "giving up" the therapist to the group. The therapist can guard against this by continually reinforcing the preparation task of the sessions and by making regular reference to how the issues can be applied in the early stages of the group.

In addition to serving as an orientation to the group, pregroup meetings can be effectively used to begin the process of establishing a therapeutic focus. This is an important priming function that facilitates the rapid emergence of a working atmosphere in the group. This can be specifically reinforced by suggesting to the patient that it would be useful, early in the group, to review such discussions with the other members. This work orientation can be the vehicle for initial self-disclosure and universality.

The two approaches, group and individual, are not mutually exclusive. A sensible combination could begin with several individual sessions under the guise of assessment, but increasingly concerned with defining a therapeutic focus. This might then be followed by a single pretherapy group session in which structured exercises are used, along with a review of the content summarized in the Appendix. It is important for the therapist conducting the preparation to clarify that it is a warm-up session and that when the therapy begins the therapist will be less active.

Preparation for group should always be considered. In some situations, for example an inpatient group, it may be adequately handled through a brief talk with the patient rather than a more formal procedure. In outpatient settings, the preparation material can be inserted into assessment interviews. The important point is to make sure the material is covered in one way or another.

Planning for the First Session

This section may seem like an exercise in the obvious. But in the rush and anxiety over beginning a group, it is not at all uncommon for mundane details to get lost. Make sure that there is absolute clarity regarding the exact date, time, and place of the first session. This is best written down and read over with the patient. There needs to be an unambiguous description of exactly where the patient should report, how to get there, where to park, and any other practical details. The time should not only be clearly spelled out but reinforced with the idea that arriving a bit early for the first session would be a good idea just in case there are any transportation snags. Similarly, be sure that arrangements have been made for doors to be unlocked, receptionists to know who to expect, and the room to be available 15 minutes before the group is to start. Consent forms and any discussion about observation or taping arrangements are best taken care of in advance. Indeed, it is nice to hold the pregroup preparation session in the group room itself and take the members through the observation room or show them how the equipment works. They may even try using the camera themselves, an exercise that helps to promote an objective perspective.

The information sheet shown in the Appendix contains the information of most value for pretherapy preparation. It can be given to the patient to take home and then be discussed in the preparation session. It should not simply be given out to be read. By spending some time with the patient going over each paragraph, an opportunity is allowed for questions or clarifications. Most critically, this reinforces the importance of the issues.

Summary

Careful thought about composing a group will assist the development of a positive working atmosphere. For time-limited group psychotherapy, some dimension of homogeneity is helpful. Within the range of homogeneity, seek as much interactional variety as possible. Systematic pretherapy preparation will help to minimize early group dropouts and will contribute to the emergence of constructive group norms. The process of thinking through composition and preparation issues also ensures that the therapist enters the group with a good understanding of each patient.

Appendix. Patient information handout

Information About Group Therapy

This information sheet is intended for patients who are about to begin group therapy, or who are considering it as a possible treatment. It is useful for people starting group therapy to have some general ideas about how groups help people and how they, themselves, can get the most out of the experience. Group therapy is different from individual therapy because many of the helpful events take place between the members and not just between the leader and the members. That is one reason why it is important that all of the members have a general introduction before beginning. Please read this material carefully and feel free to discuss any part of it with your therapist. The issues raised in this handout are also useful to talk about during the first few sessions in the group.

Do Groups Really Help People?

Group therapy is widely used and has been a standard part of treatment programs for the last 30 to 40 years. Sometimes it is used as the main or perhaps the only treatment approach. This is especially true for outpatients. Sometimes it is used as part of a treatment approach that may include individual therapy, drugs, and other activities. Group therapy has been shown in research studies to be an effective treatment. Studies that have compared individual and group approaches indicate that both are about equally effective. The difference with groups, of course, is that a group has to form, and the members need to get to know each other a bit before it can be of the greatest benefit. Most people have participated in some types of nontherapy groups, for example in schools, churches, or community activities. Therapy groups will have many of the same features. The difference is that in a therapy group the leader has a responsibility to ensure that the group stays focused on its treatment goals and that all members participate in this.

How Group Therapy Works

Group therapy is based on the idea that a great many of the difficulties that people have in their lives can be understood as problems in getting along with other people. As children, we learn ways of getting close and talking to others and ways of solving issues with others. In general, these early patterns are then applied in adult relationships. Sometimes these ways are not as effective as they might be, despite good intentions. Groups offer an opportunity to learn more about these "interpersonal" patterns. Very often, symptoms such as anxiety or unhappiness, bad feelings about yourself, or a general sense of dissatisfaction with life reflect the unsatisfactory state of important relationships. Groups are designed to help particularly with these sorts of problems. Other treatment approaches might help in other ways.

Common Myths About Group Therapy

- Although it is true that groups offer an efficient way of treating several people at once, group therapy is not a cheaper or second-rate treatment in the sense that it has less power to help people than other treatments. As mentioned above, studies show that many of the "talking therapies" are about equally effective.
- Some people are concerned that a therapy group will be like a forced confessional where they have to reveal all of the details of their lives. This is not the case. Groups will progress at their own rate as the members become more familiar with each other and can trust each other. In general, groups talk about the patterns in relationships and the meanings these have for them. For this, it is often not necessary to know specific details. Members will find their own level of comfort regarding how much they want to disclose about their personal lives. Details about where you live or work, even your last name, are not necessary for effective involvement in the group.
- Some people worry that being in a room with other people with difficulties will make everyone worse. This idea of "the blind leading the blind" is understandable, but in practice, people find that the process of talking about their problems is very helpful. Indeed, finding that others have had similar problems can be reassuring. Many group therapy patients are surprised to find that they have something to offer other people.
- Some of the media presentation of groups suggests that people will lose control in groups and become so upset they cannot function or maybe get so angry that they will be destructive. Very seldom is there any chance of this happening, and the group therapist will be alert and responsible to encourage the group if it gets too slow or to dampen things down if the tension gets too high.
- When people picture being in a therapy group, they sometimes find themselves concerned that they may be rejected or excluded by the other group members; sometimes the fear is that they will be judged

harshly by the other members, and sometimes they are afraid that they may lose their sense of themselves and be carried along by the group where they don't wish to go. All of these fears are perfectly understandable, and indeed, almost everyone experiences them to some extent when they enter a new social group situation. It is good to talk about these sorts of fears early in the group so that they can be understood and then put behind you.

How to Get the Most Out of Group Therapy

- The more you can involve yourself in the group, the more you will get out of it. In particular, try to identify the sorts of things that you find upsetting or bothersome. Try to be as open and honest as possible in what you say. Group time is precious; it is a place to be working on serious issues, not just passing the time of day. Listen hard to what people are saying, think through what they mean, and try to make sense of it. You can help others by letting them know what you make of what they say and how it affects you. Many of the issues talked about in groups are general human matters with which we can all identify. At the same time, listen hard to what others say to you about your part in the group. This process of learning from others is an important way to gain from the group experience.

- One way of thinking about group is to view it as a "living laboratory" of relationships. It is a place where you can try out new ways of talking to people, a place to take some risks. You are a responsible member of the group and can help to make it an effective experience for everybody. A good way to think about how a group can help people is this: Consider a person risking a different way of talking about personal matters, getting some response from the other members that it sounds all right, and then trying to make sense of the experience.

- Do your best to translate your inner reactions into words. Group is not a "tea party" where everything has to be done in a socially proper fashion. It is a place to try to explore the meaning of what goes on and the reactions inside that get stirred up.

- Remember that how people talk is as important as what they say. As you listen to others and as you think about what you yourself have been saying, try to think beyond the words to the other messages being sent. Sometimes the meaning of the words does not match the tone of voice or the expression on the face.

- Because the group is a place to learn from the experience itself, it is important to focus on what is happening inside the group room between the members and between each member and the leader. Often, understanding these relationships throws new light on outside relationships. Many people have found it helpful to think about themselves in terms of the things they know and don't know about themselves, and the things that others know or don't know. The diagram below outlines this. One of the tasks in group is to try to make the box called *public knowledge* larger by three main methods: 1) talk about things that you normally keep hidden about yourself or speak about your thoughts concerning others (self-disclosure), 2) listen to what others are saying about what might be your blind spots (feedback), and 3) listen hard and think hard so that you can understand more about yourself (insight).

Common Stumbling Blocks

- It is normal to feel anxious about being in groups. Almost everyone experiences it to some extent. One way of dealing with this is to talk about it at an early point in the group. This is a good model of the usefulness of talking about things so that they can be clarified and the anxiety related to them reduced.
- It is the role of the leader to encourage members to talk with each other and to help keep the group focused on important tasks. The leader is not there to supply ready answers to specific problems.

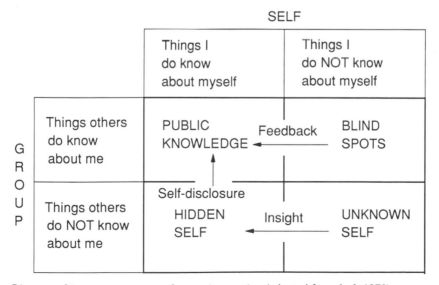

Diagram of important aspects of group interaction (adapted from Luft 1970).

One of the things you will experience in group is learning to benefit from the process of talking with other people and not just getting pat answers.

- Try hard to put into words the connection between how you are reacting or feeling and what is happening between you and other people both in the group and outside. It is all right to be emotional. This process of trying to understand reactions or symptoms in terms of relationships is important.
- Many group members find themselves experiencing a sense of puzzlement or discouragement after the excitement of the first few group sessions. Please stick with it through this stage. It almost always occurs, and it reflects the fact that it always takes groups some time to develop their full benefit for the members. Once the group has experienced this, it is in a much stronger position to be helpful.
- From time to time in the group, you may find yourself having negative feelings of disappointment, frustration, or even anger. It is important to talk about these reactions in a constructive fashion. Many people have difficulty with managing these sorts of feelings, and it is part of the group's task to examine them. Sometimes these negative feelings may be toward the leader. It is equally important that these also be talked about.
- Try hard to apply what you learn in group to outside situations. Many group members have found it very useful to talk to the group about how they might go about applying what they are learning, then try it outside in their personal lives and report back to the group about how it went. Studies have shown that the more you can do this, the more therapy becomes "real" and the more you will get out of it. At the same time, remember that the rest of the world does not necessarily run the same way as a therapy group. Try out your ideas in the group first to test if your plans are well thought out.

Group Rules

- **Confidentiality.** It is very important that things that are talked about in the group are not repeated outside. You may, of course, want to discuss your experience with people close to you but even then it is important not to attach names or specific information to the talk. In our experience, it is extremely uncommon for there to be any important break in confidentiality in therapy groups. Please be sure that you don't talk about others, just as you don't want them to talk about you outside the group.

- **Attendance and punctuality.** It is very important that you attend all sessions and arrive on time. Once a group gets going, it functions as a group, and even if just one member is absent, it is not the same. So both for your sake and for the sake of all of the members, please be a regular attendee. If for some reason it is impossible for you to make a session, then call in advance and discuss it with your therapist or at least leave the information. Then the group will know you are not coming and won't wait until you arrive to get down to work. For outpatient groups, it is useful for the group to spend some time periodically talking about major absences such as trips or vacations and discussing how to plan for these as a group.

- **Initial commitment.** Most outpatient groups meet for at least a few months. The exact number of sessions will vary according to the clinical judgment of your leader. It takes time to appreciate how much a group can help you, so it is important that you commit yourself to at least a dozen sessions of the group and that you discuss with your therapist before the group starts what the expectations are in terms of the length of your particular group.

- **Alcohol or drugs.** Groups are places for sensitive personal discussions. It is important that you do not come to sessions under the influence of alcohol or drugs except prescription medicines. This is not to say that it is good or bad to use alcohol or drugs, but they get in the way of making the most of the group experience. As a general rule, you will be asked to leave the session if your behavior is significantly affected. No food, drinks, or smoking is allowed in the group room. These tend to be distractions from the work of the group.

- **Socializing with group members.** It is important to think of groups as being a treatment setting and not as a replacement for other social activities. Group members are strongly advised not to have outside contacts with each other. The reason for this is that if you have a special relationship with another group member, that relationship gets in the way of getting the most out of the group interaction. The two of you would find yourselves having secrets from the group or not addressing issues because of your friendship. If you should have some outside contact with group members, then it is important that this be talked about in the group so that the effects can be taken into account. You are asked to make a commitment to report such contacts within the group.

- **Major life decisions.** Many people come to therapy groups because things have not been going well in their lives. There is a temptation to take the first advice you hear and decide to make a big change. Please wait so that you have a chance to get the most out of your therapy before making important life decisions.

CHAPTER 8

The Beginning

This chapter applies the group theories discussed in Section I to a beginning psychotherapy group. The management of the first session is a critical time because this is where the tone of the therapy is set. Methods for addressing the two major tasks of stage 1—developing cohesion and defining the external group boundary—are described. Techniques for maximizing the effects of therapeutic factors are presented as well as some of the practicalities of group management. Issues relating to individual members and the social roles they play are considered. In this and succeeding chapters, examples are drawn from a variety of actual group experiences.

The First Session

Care taken in preparation for the first session will be well repaid. Not infrequently, last-minute arrangements have to be made. Details for including a final member have to be completed. A potential member telephones at the last minute with vague questions about when the group should start or ambivalence about coming. The therapist may well be experiencing some natural anxiety over how the group is going to begin. In short, it is a time fraught with the potential for minor problems.

One might liken the first session of a group to the first few minutes of a play. You may not know where the plot is going to lead, you might not have met all of the characters, but you quickly begin to get a clear sense of the firmness of the production and the care with which it has been put together. The same thoughts apply to the first group session.

The Room

Be sure the room is set up in advance. It does not make a good impression to walk into a room that has just been vacated by a family with a hyperactive child and find it a scene of chaos. Chairs should be set up in a reasonably tight circle with one chair for each member, no more and no less. If possible, avoid long sofas that cluster members and may interfere with each member having a clear view of all others. In general, it is preferable not to have a table within the circle. Tables invite the depositing of books, cups, clothing, feet, and anything else that can serve as a barrier. An open space sends a clear message that talking to each other is the purpose. If a table is present, it must be low. The room should be well lit though not glaring. Subdued lights in a group room suggest secrecy and internal reflection, not self-disclosure and interaction. If audiovisual equipment is to be used, it should be tested and set up and ready to go with only the Pause button waiting to be released.

There are some advantages to having the group members assemble in a waiting area and then move to the group room together a few minutes before the starting time. The therapist then joins them on time if all are present or after a very brief delay if all are not there. This approach is designed to focus on the role of the leader and avoid contamination with social niceties.

Carefully close the door, even if some group members have not arrived. This is a powerful symbolic statement regarding the external group boundary. It avoids the indecision of expectant, perhaps pleading glances toward the outside, awaiting the arrival of any additional members. To latecomers, it is an implicit message regarding time boundaries. To those in the room, it reinforces their promptness and indicates that the group is going to work with whomever is present. These structural issues are designed to create a "frame" around the therapeutic experience. This helps to clarify what is inside the group and what is outside.

Careful adherence to these ideas fosters the impression of a well-organized and professional atmosphere in which important work is anticipated. It does not mean that pleasantness or humanness is abandoned, but that there are clear structural expectations regarding the process of group participation. This allows the members to relax in the knowledge that they are in good hands.

Beginning the First Session

Members will anticipate that the group is going to be conducted by the therapist. This is not an unrealistic expectation if they have not previously been in a therapy situation. Remember that in assessment interviews the major responsibility for the production of information has come from the interviewer, with the patient in a responding mode. Pretherapy preparation will not alter the hope and expectation that the real responsibility will continue to lie with the therapist.

The task of the therapist is an inherently contradictory one: to facilitate group interaction without taking over or inhibiting group initiative. The technical question is how best to accomplish this. The importance of group-initiated actions should be stressed in the pretherapy period, referred to in the opening sessions, and reinforced at all opportunities. However, it is also appropriate for the therapist to take some initiative if the group is reluctant to do so.

This may be an issue of controversy with some therapists. They would argue that bad habits should not be fostered and the members must realize from the onset that the therapist is not going to initiate. However, prolonged silence or trivial conversation in the first session can be counterproductive. It is preferable that the group address its therapeutic task early even if this entails the therapist providing some modest structure around which this can occur. Even while using the structure, the therapist may offer interpretive comments to the effect that this is not a pattern that will continue forever and that it is understood that members will be eager to take the initiative.

If members have never been in the therapy room, a few minutes may be taken to review its contents. This might also be a time to reinforce the idea of no drinks, food, or smoking. If audiovisual equipment is being used, whether it be a simple audio recording within the room, video cameras, or observation windows, these should be openly described and identified. Although it is useful to have such equipment as inconspicuous as possible, it should not be hidden. It is better to directly acknowledge the presence and location of equipment in order to desensitize the members to any sense of mystery or secrecy regarding it. This is also an opportunity to reiterate issues of confidentiality by reviewing how tapes will be handled.

Introductions

The first interactional task is to make introductions. Usually at this point, some members are eager to get the ball rolling. If so, the therapist can immediately back out of the group interaction and let the group members take on the task of getting to know each other. A brief reminder might be inserted during this process to the effect that personal details concerning last names, employment, or area of residence are not important in the group and need not be disclosed. The group is to work on problems within the room in confidentiality, and specific details about outside life circumstances are unnecessary.

Allowing members to begin structuring the group process illustrates a general principle—group therapy must be considered not just as therapy in a group, but therapy by the group. From within the resources of the membership, groups are generally able to provide an endless richness of therapeutic experiences. In a very real sense, the challenge to the leader is to avoid interfering with that process.

It is not unusual for the first go-around to consist of a rapid identification by first name followed by silence. It is useful for the therapist to immediately deepen the experience by acknowledging everyone's participation, perhaps reflecting the sense of understandable anxiety in the occasion, and wondering if members could talk more in a general way about the sorts of issues that they would like to address in the group. This is the point where the work of preliminary sessions will have its rewards. It quickly establishes the norm within the group that serious personal issues will be the main subject of the group's activity. The central point is not that this work focus is conducted at a profound level of insight, but rather the implicit acknowledgment that the group is to be used for constructive work. Members can be expected to react to this with an attempt to lighten the atmosphere or retreat back to social amenities. Such a reaction is best quickly addressed by identifying the process and reiterating the task. The style with which this is done must be carefully judged. It must not come across as criticism, but rather as encouragement to get at a difficult job.

Latecomers

There are often latecomers to first sessions. It is useful to think through specific ways of addressing their arrival. Not infrequently, such an event constitutes the first evidence of ambivalence about the group task or resistance toward the organizational approach as it has been set up by the leader. The therapist may be inclined to address these resistive features of tardiness as an initial demonstration of professional acumen. But this is not the time for such interpretations. It is preferable to provide a positive example of norm establishment without invoking comments that might be taken as criticism or blame. One approach might be to greet and seat the member and indicate that there will be a chance to get introduced to the group once the present topic of discussion has come to a natural point of closure. In terms of operant conditioning, this does not reinforce a grand entrance with attention. The point may be reiterated at the end of the session by stressing for the entire membership the importance of beginning on time so that the group indeed can function as a group.

Norm Reinforcement

It is useful to specifically reinforce the basic group "rules" before the session ends. Hopefully these have already been covered in pretherapy sessions. They should be briefly but explicitly restated with an invitation for any further response or elaboration from the members regarding them. Usually there are plenty of opportunities to slip such material into the ongoing group conversation.

A particularly pertinent topic is that of extragroup socializing, because this becomes an immediate possibility at the end of the first session. Many groups go for coffee after the session. It is not possible for the therapist to absolutely govern this, nor need it necessarily be a harmful process. It may provide a forum through which the group can offer a significant amount of support. The therapist does need to underline the reasons for concerns about extragroup socializing. In particular, it should be stressed that the group should be informed of any such activities. It is also useful to review what the implications are of some members going for coffee but not others. These comments are not meant to condone extragroup socializing; however, there are realistic limits to what can be controlled, and an overly stringent approach can create a climate of authoritarian control that may interfere later.

Process Debriefing

Before the group ends, it is very helpful to elicit comments from all members concerning their reaction to the first session. These are almost always positive and serve to reinforce cohesion. However, the exercise may also flush out negative or ambivalent positions that need to be addressed. Usually, a lack of enthusiasm is based on untested assumptions about what will happen or misunderstandings of some aspects of the session. Opening these up for discussion usually serves to defuse them. Such topics will also draw in other members as group supporters, which reinforces their commitment to the group and may provide an opportunity for altruistic behavior.

At a deeper level, by drawing attention to the process, the therapist is setting a good model for addressing issues promptly, calmly, and fearlessly even if they are not entirely of a positive nature. The group is being molded into thinking about process events, a task that will continue throughout its life.

New therapists should take solace from the fact that the first session of a group is almost always a roaring success. The members are even more anxious than the therapist and will work hard to make it a productive occasion. The initial self-revelations are deeply felt and produce both relief and a sense of membership. In the best of worlds, the therapist may need to do very little but let these processes flow. Under more difficult circumstances, there may be the need for greater activity in encouraging the sorts of dimensions that will be most productive for the early group.

Reference was made in the preceding discussion to building norm development comments onto issues raised by the members. This is a very important therapeutic technique. The therapist should go into the first session, indeed every session, with a short agenda of items that need to be covered at some point. Almost invariably, if the matter is important to the therapist, some member has also developed the same idea. The therapist can wait for a reasonable opportunity and build reinforcing or focusing statements onto a part of the ongoing group interaction. This serves to validate the group's sense of its own potential for work and reduces the profile of leader control.

Basic Tasks

The primary group task of stage 1 is to resolve the question of membership. This task will extend over numerous sessions. The group must come out of this stage with a committed group of members. In this process, it is not uncommon for one or two members to be lost. Commitment to the work of the group is reflected in a strong sense of group identity and a well-defined external group boundary.

Developing Cohesion

The principal responsibility of the therapist during the first few sessions is to the development of the group system, not to the individual members. The development and maintenance of group cohesion forms the central task. It is essential that a sense of positive identification with the group emerge at an early point. Otherwise, demoralization will set in, with disenchantment over the possibilities of group psychotherapy, and diminishing motivation to participate actively. This may lead to premature terminations that further undermine belief in the group and can escalate into group disintegration. Fortunately, as mentioned in Chapter 2, there is a strong tendency for group members to view their own group in positive terms, to strive for a sense of homogeneity within the group, and to see outside groups in critical terms. This natural desire for a positive group experience is a powerful motivator.

The therapist must make sure that all members participate in this initial work. At the same time, the first stage should not be unnecessarily prolonged. Pretherapy preparation and a degree of homogeneity assist the engagement process. Time is of particular concern in brief groups in which perseveration in the positive environment of early group phenomena may shorten the time left for more challenging and confronting activities. Therefore, for very pragmatic reasons, the therapist must have a primary concern for how the group is coalescing.

The concept of the *working alliance* was discussed in Chapter 2 as an important predictor of positive outcome in individual therapy. A major advantage in groups is that the working alliance is enacted between the members and is not solely dependent on the relationship with the therapist. Thus, a group that develops a cohesive atmosphere has a broader base for sustaining support. Negative factors that might interfere with cohesion in the early group need to be dealt with promptly and thoroughly. Ways of addressing such issues are discussed later in this chapter.

Promoting interaction among members.   One powerful method for enhancing cohesion is to specifically promote member-to-member interaction. By encouraging members to talk with each other, bonds between them will be automatically created. This is a simple therapeutic technique, which involves continuous scanning of the directionality of group interaction and gently guiding it. The most common problem is a tendency for members to want to talk to or through the therapist. The leader should be comfortable in specifically redirecting comments. Such phrases might be tried as, "Perhaps you might want to see what Walter thinks about that idea; it sounds like something he was saying earlier," or "It is important that everyone in the group get to know how the others understand things—Why don't you try that out on someone else." Such interventions will not appear avoidant or too controlling if the rationale has been established during pretherapy preparation that intermember activity is an important component to the group therapeutic experience. Directional structuring activities make explicit the message that members are going to be of help to each other. The therapist may specifically break eye contact as it is established with one member and look directly at other group members as a nonverbal reinforcement to promote member interaction. Such covert interventions should generally be used along with direct comments about the value of member-to-member interchanges.

Sometimes a few active members dominate the group interaction by talking to each other. The therapist will need to bring in other members to ensure that all participate. This is not unexpected and should be handled directly and openly as a necessary task to be sure that all group members benefit. The therapist might make a comment such as, "Well, Marsha and Scott, you two have had a good chance to get into some important issues. I guess we need to hear about some of the matters that others have on their minds. We'll get back to your concerns later. Bea, you looked like you were going to say something a few minutes ago." It is of particular importance that all members participate in the first session. This diffuses anxiety about future sessions and also consolidates identification with the group.

Creating a therapeutic milieu.   The therapist can help the group by promoting an environment in which therapeutic factors from the supportive cluster can flourish. Such a group climate is characterized by a positive and supportive quality with concern for individual distress. This empathic stance facilitates open and trusting exchanges. As these develop, the group will come to assume increasing importance in the psychological life of the members. They will find themselves thinking about past sessions and about what they want to say in the next session. This reflective process should be encouraged and used as part of group work. The group comes to be viewed as an important function that offers hope that personal problems can be usefully addressed. Members also learn that they can be of value to each other. This altruistic experience reinforces self-esteem. There is increasing use of the term *we* to refer to the group, as members experience higher levels of acceptance from others.

Some technical characteristics of a therapeutic culture that need to be reinforced include spontaneity, a willingness to speak up at once with ideas, and asking for clarification if unsure what a person means. Members can be urged to listen carefully to others and to monitor their own reactions. Comments addressed to specific other members should be encouraged. The therapist can ask that general comments about the group be clarified by specific examples: "Howie, you mentioned that you found the session helpful. What was it particularly that helped? Can you tell us what was the most important point in the session for you?" Rapid changes of topic should be discouraged, although undue length in any one area may become sterile. Above all, the members need to feel that they themselves have some responsibility for the process of change.

Self-disclosure, interpersonal challenge, and introspective understanding may be in evidence, but at a relatively superficial level. The therapist should be careful not to push such mechanisms too vigorously until the group has developed adequate cohesion. Conflict and confrontation between members is usually low in early sessions, although at a later time, group members may acknowledge that they had been aware of issues that were avoided. The therapist may gently dampen negative dimensions while implying that they will form suitable work for the group a bit later.

Defining the External Boundary

In the engagement stage, the external group boundary must be defined. This idea of boundary clarification can be addressed in a systematic manner. The therapist may use techniques that promote exploration of issues that will assist in focusing on the boundary. In its simplest terms, this means an investigation of things that are unique within the group compared with outside relationship experiences.

The physical boundary. The importance of beginning the first session of the group in a clear and unambiguous fashion has already been mentioned. By seating the group members in a special room, entering as the designated leader, and closing the door, the therapist has begun the process of defining the group's external boundary. These actions say louder than words that we are in this together and must sort out how we as a group are going to operate.

It is highly desirable to have the group meet in the same room under the same conditions for each session. For example, if a group is to be observed, it should meet systematically in the observation room even if on some occasions no observers are present. Changes in the time the group meets should be made very carefully as well. Shifting the time schedule to accommodate a member or the leader implies a violation of the original contract and thus weakens the external boundary.

The membership boundary.   The question of membership speaks directly to the heart of external boundary definition. Early in the group's life, the therapist must be constantly aware of the impact of changes of membership as a result of repeated absences or premature terminations. Such issues cannot be brushed under the carpet with a rationale that they will get sorted out later. They are fundamental to the definition of the group and must be addressed and resolved. A member, for example, who misses several of the first six sessions of a group must be directly confronted with the issue of membership. Confrontation does not mean that the behavior is addressed in a punitive fashion. There may be perfectly understandable reasons why the member cannot attend. For whatever reason, if attendance is going to be sporadic, then it is in the best interest of the group that the member be guided into an alternative therapeutic program. This is one specific example of the therapist acting on behalf of the group, not the individual, during the first stage.

If observers sit in the group room, as sometimes happens in educational institutions, then it should be clearly understood that any given observer must attend regularly for a specific duration. Laxity in such issues sends a message to the group that the external boundary of the group is inconstant and therefore that they themselves also do not need to take it seriously.

The time boundary.   There should be no ambiguity concerning when the group starts and ends. The clear expectation is that all members come on time and leave only at the end. As with attendance, members who cannot do this should be placed elsewhere. Groups should begin on time, even if all members are not present. They should also end on time. Only in extremely unusual situations should the ending time be extended. Such a practice invites members to delay bringing up important matters and thus win extra group time and attention. The group cannot substitute for real-life circumstances, and one aspect of this is the necessity of facing the "real world" on time.

An overly accommodating approach to time boundaries suggests that the interests of those who are attending regularly and on time are being sacrificed. This is not an issue of compulsivity or punitiveness. A group can be a group only when its members are present. The absence of even one member makes a difference in how the group operates. Altering either the beginning or ending time provides circumstances in which all members may not be able to participate.

The information boundary.   Another major mechanism at work in the engagement stage is a process of comparing experiences in the group with those that members have had outside of the group. This creates an implicit recognition that there is an information boundary. The process of universalization creates a sense of what the inside of the group is about and therefore allows comparisons with other groups. This information about differences helps to consolidate a sense of groupness. Generally speaking, members coming to psychotherapy groups have experienced adverse issues in their current or past relationships. Almost always, the early group experiences are infused with an atmosphere of positive excitement. It is therefore easy to contrast them with outside experiences. This should not be done by encouraging critical language that may reinforce the patient's misperceptions or distortions regarding such outside experiences. Rather, the emphasis should be on the occurrence of positive experiences within the group. For example, "You describe problems in talking openly with your wife, but it seems very constructive that you have been able to open up about these important personal issues here in the group," or "It sounds like letting some of those pent-up emotions come out in the group is a different way for you, but that may be of value in your outside relationships in which you keep things locked up inside." Using the guideline of in-out differences, the therapist can systematically reinforce the external group boundary. Therapy is more effective when attention is devoted to the application of therapeutic experiences to outside circumstances and relationships. The presence of a clearly understood external boundary assists this process because it highlights ways in which the two experiences differ or are the same. This promotes the use of finer distinctions in how to apply therapy learning to the world outside.

Once a group is well established with a sustained cohesive atmosphere, minor lapses in the above boundary issues can be tolerated. However, in the early sessions they constitute an important mechanism for assisting the formation of a sense of groupness. We shall see in Chapter 11 that many of the same principles apply during termination work.

Therapeutic Strategies

Using Therapeutic Factors

The therapeutic factors that are of most value to the group in stage 1 are drawn primarily from the supportive and self-revelation clusters. The therapist can systematically reinforce their contribution to the task of engagement.

Hope.   The presence of this factor will have been felt from the first pretherapy interview, actually from the first telephone call to make an appointment. In the group, it will be reinforced by the opportunity to talk about important personal issues and experience a positive reception to them.

Acceptance.   The experience of becoming part of a group constitutes a powerful validation of the self. The sense of belongingness is a powerful reinforcement of group participation. Many patients coming for therapy experience themselves as on the outside of "normal" society and view their need for help with shame. In a therapy group, the opposite is the case. The decision to seek therapy is viewed not only as positive, but as an indication of strength. The therapist can facilitate this factor by making sure that every patient participates to some extent in every session.

Each sensitive or delicate issue raised requires a response from others. Highly charged statements should not be met with silence. Sometimes patients will slip in statements regarding events in their lives without any elaboration. These may relate to some major event such as a family death or a traumatic rape. If the factual information is dissociated from the affect, the members may politely let it pass without comment. The therapist must engineer a response if none is forthcoming. Any reasonably positive response will augment the patient's sense of acceptance and normalize the distress being described.

Altruism. The self-disclosure statements made early in a group place responsibility on other group members for a validating response. Members become, in a sense, responsible for the well-being of their peers. This experience of altruism, of being of help to others, is highly motivating and contributes to group cohesion. It also makes the giver feel good. This is a paradoxical situation in which the person coming for help experiences enhancement of self-esteem through helping others. The mechanism of altruism is seldom found in individual psychotherapy but can be specifically promoted and explored in the group context.

Self-revelation. Early group sessions depend on the self-revelation factors of self-disclosure and catharsis. Pretherapy sessions will have stressed the importance of revealing internal thoughts and taking some risks in the group. The process of actually putting personally important material into words in a group is experienced as quite arousing and threatening. It is a necessary precursor for universality.

The content of early disclosures is usually of a factual nature. The material is important, not for psychological understanding, but as an opportunity to identify with other members. The therapist therefore should not explore the significance of such self-disclosure too vigorously. The less comfortable work of the therapy is best conducted later, with a base of support and sense of safety. However, the therapist can actively work to mold the nature of self-disclosure so that it is primarily centered around psychological material that will be of value for later work. Lengthy factual discourses with many specific details are less relevant than information about the meaning of experiences and nature of reactions. The therapist has to walk a delicate line between shaping the material in the service of group interactional norms and shutting down participation in the process. This is sometimes effectively handled by referring to other members with similar problems in whom the relationship meanings can be more easily underlined.

An important component of the self-disclosure process is to risk putting sensitive problems into words and then experience a response that is different from that expected. Members will be extremely alert to the reaction of others when they say something of personal importance. The therapist must recognize the power of these experiences and the need to ensure that a positive result emerges. The nature of the response of other members should be carefully monitored. In the great majority of cases, members will respond in an understanding and supportive fashion to the disclosure of almost anything. The therapist can ensure that these reactions are put into words and that the individual hears those words. In a sense, the therapist can conduct an "instant replay" of the process with the addition of commentary. For example, "What you have just said sounds like it is an important issue for you. Did you understand what Jo was saying about it? Jo, do you want to repeat what you said to be sure that Cecil understands how you feel?" This *massaging of the process* is a technique that will be used in many situations. Risking a personally important statement and experiencing a positive response from other group members can be a powerful experience. It not only indicates that the member is becoming accepted by the group, it also serves as personal validation that enhances self-esteem.

Universality.   The most pervasive mechanism for the development of engagement is universality—the recognition that others in the group have had experiences similar to one's own. This process forms the seed around which a sense of group identity can develop. It creates the content that comes to represent the group and helps to define its external boundary. This is the experience that can be compared and contrasted with life outside the group. Universality thus fosters an appreciation of the group as a unique entity. As groups begin their first interactions, a process of searching for common experiences, common symptoms, and common personal reactions takes place. Efforts to use some homogeneous criteria in group composition will now be rewarded.

      The experience of universality contributes to a lowering of social anxiety. It is often accompanied by a sense of exhilaration sometimes close to euphoria. This process of searching for sameness typically involves an uncritical acceptance of information about others in which ambiguity and rapid assumptions go unchallenged. Generally in psychotherapy groups, the content of universality centers around symptoms such as depression or anxiety, stress experiences such as bereavement or separation, and descriptors of self such as low self-esteem. All of these constitute aspects of the "human condition." They are important in a therapy group first because they create a common focus and second because they are related to psychological issues. They form a base from which more complex understanding can develop. In early group sessions, they are primarily important because they are a vehicle for creating a general sense of universality. It is this component that the therapist needs to reinforce. Simple bridging statements can be used, such as, "It sounds to me, Rae, that you have had several experiences that are very parallel to those that Ruth was talking about last week." Universality can be pushed further with process encouragement: "Your reaction to your divorce sounds similar to Diane's reaction to the death of her mother. Could the two of you explore further what those experiences were like?" The important issue for the therapist to keep in mind during the early group sessions is that it is the process of finding similarities that is of most value to the group. This is not the time for exploration into personal depth but rather for the revelation of information that will promote mutual identification. One can feel comfortable with, and have the illusion of understanding, someone who has had similar experiences.

The therapeutic technique that flows from this is a simple one. It consists of clarification interventions that will result in the elaboration of content themes that can be linked among the members. At the same time, the therapist may be keeping careful track of important issues being raised by each member for future exploration, but the task initially is group formation.

Task focus.   Cohesion can also be reinforced through recognition of the importance of the psychotherapeutic task. As relevant issues are brought to the fore, the therapist should specifically relate these to the task of resolving specific problems. This builds on the assessment and pretherapy preparation process. Systematic reinforcement of comments relating to psychological goals or problem identification helps to develop the working alliance. Although the specifics will be unique to each individual, the importance of task focus with its implicit recognition of the need for change is an important common factor.

Negative reactions.   The therapist needs to be alert to the emergence of themes of conflict, criticism, or rejection. In general, these do not arise during early sessions, but when they do, they need to be skillfully handled by the therapist. Usually, drawing attention to a positive component and shifting the focus is adequate. Try to find evidence of universality that can be reinforced. At times, the therapist may need to temporarily take over control of the process and request that conflictual material be delayed until a later point in the group's life: "I can understand that it must be difficult for you to understand Maureen's experience (*initial alignment*). Both of you seem to have had pretty upsetting times in your marriages (*universality*). As we get to know each other better in here, we will have an opportunity to get further into those things (*suitable to talk about but not now*). Let's put it on hold for now and see what others have on their minds (*unambiguous control*)." The emergence of high levels of conflict in the first few sessions correlates with premature terminations and with groups that fail to progress. Patients beginning psychotherapy are generally particularly sensitive to judgmental issues, and the strength of negative comments will be amplified severalfold because of the perception that they reflect a general group opinion. Usually, some group members will intervene quickly if such material escalates, but the therapist has a clear responsibility to step in if the level of negative affect rises too much.

Therapist Style and Technique

Another mechanism for defining the external group boundary is the common identification of the group members with the therapist. This hearkens back to Freud's idea that in groups the members are tied together through their common projection of internal issues onto the leader. In the early group, this common identification is primarily seen in statements of exaggerated appreciation of the power and wisdom of the leader. In informational terms, the leader is the only person in the room with a clearly identified role and professional responsibilities. Members will identify not only with each other and their similarities but also as members of "Dr. So-and-So's Group." It is best not to seriously challenge unrealistic assumptions early on, until the group has more cohesion. As discussed above, the process can be usefully begun by promoting intermember interaction and striving to decrease the amount of time spent talking to the leader. Personally, the leader should bear in mind that the effusion of positive remarks is in part promoted by group necessity and therefore needs to be taken with a grain of salt.

Leader Task

The leader must attend not to individual psychodynamic issues, but to the process of commitment to the group. Responsibility is toward the new group system more than to the individual members. The group can be assisted in its task by encouraging and reinforcing supportive cluster factors, especially universality and inside/outside comparisons. Early self-disclosure should be reinforced, and its superficial nature be allowed to pass without comment. There will be a strong tendency for members to look toward the leader for solutions and helpful hints. Such requests are normal and need to be handled with tact, not abrupt denial.

Activity Level

It is appropriate for the therapist to be moderately active during the first few sessions. There are some guidelines for this. The therapist is active only when necessary. Some groups move smoothly into engagement processes, and the therapist can only sit back and admire their astuteness. The thrust of therapist interventions should be to promote the sort of therapeutic dimensions discussed in this chapter. That is, they should be primarily devoted to molding group process in the service of creating a therapeutic milieu. Therapist actions should be viewed as an opportunity for modeling. Specific reference to this aspect can be made with statements like, "You may notice that I was trying to get Bob to talk about the meaning of his experience in that situation. The group may like to help each other to keep focused on this sort of question." Therapist activity should generally be in an exploratory, not a directive, style. Above all, the therapist must be prepared to gradually decrease activity level as the group gains in ability to provide its own stimulus (39).

Leader Style

The actions of the leader are carefully observed by the members and used as a model for how to participate in the group. The leader therefore must be careful about his or her group behavior and design it to provide the sort of role model that is best suited to helping the group coalesce. At a structural level, it is common in early sessions for members to automatically want to make most of their comments to the leader. This is hardly surprising, particularly if they have seen the leader alone before the group or if they have had any preceding individual therapy. The therapist might conceptualize his or her function during the early sessions primarily in positive and supportive terms. The therapist should appreciate that beginning a group is not easy and that members will respond positively to encouragement and understanding. In particular, in the early sessions, interpretive statements are seldom useful and may be understood as criticism or attack. As part of the grouping process, members want to make a positive impression. Interpretations may be seen as blocking this.

Clarification

One constructive technique is to consistently seek clarification. This may be applied to group events or to content themes. By requesting further clarification or further elaboration, the therapist is modeling a process that has powerful learning features and is at the same time encouraging members to commit themselves with further revelations to the group. It also provides a good model for group members to adopt to gain further information from each other. One useful way of doing this is to stay alert to the problem areas that were elicited from each member during assessment. By making these problems "public property" at an early point, clarification questions can be used to connect a given action or remark to these focal themes.

Process Over Content

Attention to process is more important than attention to content. This is as true in the early stages of a group as it is later. The techniques of clarification and genuine interest in the process do a great deal to promote group interaction. A powerful yet simple method is to inquire about what members thought was going on between them. By presenting such questions in a nonaccusing and noninterpretive manner, but simply out of interest, the therapist can lead the group to greater comfort in exploring process events: "You two just had a pretty serious exchange about things that are very important. Could you say a little bit about what it was like to talk in the group like that?" Often such nonintrusive methods provide rapid access to emotionally loaded issues. Technically correct interpretations may run up against defensive barriers if the group is not ready for them. The therapist should be particularly alert to pick up process events that relate to the themes discussed in this chapter. By drawing attention to these dimensions, they can be reinforced. This underlining technique is a powerful but subtle way of molding the group toward more effective work.

Group-Level Interpretations

Formal interpretations about the dynamics of the whole group generally fall on barren ground. Because the group is just in the process of forming, members will find it hard to use such metaphoric language. However, it is useful to label and to be interested in common group reactions. Often these may center around common states of anxiousness over beginning the group, common expectations about the nature of the role of the leader, and common fears about appearing silly, weak, or immature in the eyes of other members. By such clarification, these reactions are usually tempered.

The Individual Member

The development of group cohesion has been emphasized as the primary task of the therapist in stage 1. The process of making a commitment to the group has an important effect for the individual as well. This is an example of the isomorphy between group process and internal psychological events. The experience of universality—"joining the human race"—may be a powerful one. To appreciate that other people have had reactions that oneself had viewed as extreme, shameful, or sick is a powerful first step in reconceptualizing oneself. The idea of being found acceptable by others, even of helping others, may be a profound experience.

Just as important is the idea that commitment to membership is also a commitment to work. Indeed, the therapist should be sure that these two processes are regularly linked together. Agreeing to join means taking the group work seriously, but it also implies taking oneself seriously. This represents a further step on the road to personal change. Beginning to address personal issues often reflects a fundamental shift in self-perception. Therapy carries an implicit statement of self-assertion and self-valuation, not of being a passive recipient or victim. This may be combined with hopes of being rescued or magically altered, but nonetheless is an element to the early sessions that should be sought out and reinforced.

In focusing on group development, the therapist must not forget that the individual members need support from the therapist as well as from the group itself. During the final third of each session, it is useful to scan the group in terms of members who have said little or with whom there has not been a direct exchange. Somehow, they need to be included. For the member, a sense of being valued by the therapist is a powerful motivator.

The responsibility of the leader to the group more than to the individual in the early sessions has been stressed. This is meant as a guiding orientation. Of course, the therapist has a professional responsibility to the welfare of each individual as well. In a way, the duty to develop the group is cloaked in interactions directed at the individual.

However, on occasion, individuals do not seem to be taking smoothly to the group environment. There may be many reasons for this. The group composition may have created an isolate within the group. The stress of the group environment may inflame pathological impulsivity that is difficult to contain. Some people seem determined to turn the entire group against them despite all efforts of the therapist to mediate the process. And for some members, their ambivalence about the idea of therapy may become increasingly evident.

The therapist must be prepared to intervene if there appears to be the risk of a harmful experience. It is useful to remember that all of the members in a new group will be struggling as best they know how to survive and be accepted. They may lose sight of the effects of their actions on some members. In most cases, it is adequate for the therapist to simply draw attention to an area of concern and have it addressed. For example, "In all the enthusiasm to get started, Ann hasn't had a chance to get in yet. Have you found some issues today that make sense for you?" Or, "John has been an active participant today, and is sorting of getting jumped on. I wonder if he's taking the heat for some concerns that others might have as well."

Sometimes it becomes clear early on that a particular member is not going to fit in the group. This may reflect composition issues, or simply that the individual is not suited to group therapy. In these sorts of situations, it may be in the patient's best interest, as well as the group's, that a peaceful parting of the ways take place. The management of such an occurrence is challenging. It is reviewed later in this chapter under premature terminations and also in the next chapter under scapegoating.

Social Roles

During the engagement stage, role behaviors drawn from the positive side of the spectrum are particularly important, indeed essential, to group development. Thus, the sociable and structural roles appear most active.

The therapist may reinforce the positive contributions made by different types of members. This will enhance the engagement process. In this regard, the social role descriptions in Chapter 4 may be taken as a starting point. This should be done carefully, however. Each role type also carries with it liabilities that will need to be addressed eventually. Therefore, comments are best targeted at specific types of behavior and should not carry a global message that everything is satisfactory. The divergent and cautionary role representatives may need more therapist support, because the group will automatically reward its more positive contributors. Great care must be taken that certain members do not appear to be the therapist's favorites. It is easy to inadvertently get this idea across, in gratitude to some members for taking on leadership functions.

Sociable role.   The emphasis these members place on positive interactions and the involvement of all members are invaluable during the early stages of the group. Their warmth and nonthreatening approach elicit participation from others. A trusting nature often makes it easier for them to reveal important information, thus modeling self-disclosure. These members experience the early support of the group for their activities. This support and the beneficial effects of ventilation and self-disclosure may produce early symptomatic improvement. Thus, hope is reinforced for others.

The therapist can feel comfortable in allowing such members to go about their social support activities and may want to modestly encourage them in this task. However, these very qualities will at a later point provide difficulties for sociable role members. Care must be taken that they are not identified as the ideal group participant simply because what they have to offer is of particular value early in the group's life. A safer path is to encourage generalization and modeling of the behaviors they are using as an important group goal rather than focusing on them as the main providers of such input.

Structural role.   The focus of the structural role leaders on identifying problems and establishing a work ethic forms a useful model for the developing group. This complements the activity of the sociable role members in helping to develop a positive working climate. The desire of the structural role members to understand and explain behavior, rather than just to experience it like the sociable role members, exerts a calming influence on the group. It addresses the fear that group emotion will get out of hand. Generally, the structural role members are appreciated for their efforts. If they become too active, they may be seen to be interfering with the development of the group experience. At such a point, they may need some support from the therapist and encouragement to sit back and observe more than dominate.

Divergent role.   Members who represent the behaviors characteristic of the divergent role are welcomed for their enthusiastic engagement into group process. However, their emphasis on differences and confrontation works against the creation of group cohesion. The therapist needs to be attentive to the input from these members and to be prepared to reframe it in stage 1 terms without alienating or shutting down such members. Using the language of universality and the supportive factors usually accomplishes this. For example, differences expressed by a divergent role member may be interpreted as an important demonstration of people talking openly in the group. Support can be given for the issues raised and reassurance that they will be talked about eventually.

Cautionary role. These members tend to be silent observers during early sessions. Although they need to be encouraged to participate, often a small contribution goes a long way. The reluctance of cautionary role members may be translated into the importance of taking small steps in joining the group. The therapist may be reassured that these members, although of less value in addressing stage 1 issues, will be of importance later. It is important not to align with the view that those who participate at a low level are going to handicap the group.

Predictable Problems

Premature Terminations

Most premature terminations in group therapy occur in the first six sessions. Beyond that point, unpredicted terminations are infrequent and usually result from some intense event. The therapist can be reassured that it is not a catastrophe to lose a group member at an early point, though reasonable efforts need to be extended to try to forestall this from happening. The most important principle is to address directly any remarks suggesting doubt about continuing. To ignore hints about such material is to encourage it. Generally speaking, the source of such doubts is understandable but correctable. If the member does drop out, at least the matter has been addressed and is not an entirely unpredicted event. The remaining members will have some understanding of the issues, which will serve to create a rationale for the loss. Because there will be strong pressures to consolidate group integrity, these rationales are quickly accepted. In the first few sessions, relationships between members are just forming, and the departure has its greatest importance in terms of group morale, not the loss of the individual.

If group efforts are not sufficient to persuade a member to remain, the therapist should have a private discussion with the particular member after the group meeting. The task in these efforts is not to dissuade the individual from the decision but rather to understand the basis for it and to clarify issues. This may be important for the individual. Personal material not brought up in the group may cast a different light on the circumstances and an alternative referral might be helpful. In addition, a negative therapeutic experience may block future efforts at seeking help; therefore, efforts to defuse separation tension may be of value. Care should be taken that an accusatory tone is not adopted.

When a member does decide to leave a group at an early stage, some therapists insist that the person come back to a final session to "say good-bye" or to "clear up unfinished business." Such efforts are usually futile. If the individual does return, a perfunctory explanation is made, this is accepted by the group, and everyone sits around in uneasy apprehension waiting for the actual separation to occur. An exception to this is when the decision to leave is directly related to a specific group event. Some opportunity to clarify the intent or meaning of the experience may be useful both for the one departing as well as for the other group participants in it. A common reaction at an unexpected termination is for other group members, or perhaps the therapist, to feel that the circumstances were mishandled and that someone must bear responsibility for the loss. In fact, such situations almost always are complex and involve both sides of the issue. It is important that the group have an opportunity for a thorough discussion of the circumstances with or without the departing member.

This position regarding the futility of having a person come back for a final session is based on the fact that usually the person has been backing out of the group for several sessions and is not highly committed to it. Thus, the question of group relationships is not highly charged. For the other group members, the major implications are the survival of the group. It is important that the departure not get in the way of ongoing group cohesion. In the next chapter, we shall discuss the idea of the group scapegoat who is in fact acting out group tension. This is an entirely different set of issues from the early dropout who is not yet fully committed to the group.

It is useful to bear in mind that the decision to terminate therapy might be in the best interests of the individual. Dropouts may correctly sense that they are getting into dangerous territory that they will not be able to handle. They may be concerned that to continue would risk negative or unsuccessful experiences that might reinforce doubts about self-effectiveness. In short, early terminations are not uncommon and are not necessarily damaging to the individual or to the group. What is important is that the issues are openly discussed in the group so that misconceptions and individual reactions can be clarified.

Overly Intense Self-disclosure

The therapist also needs to monitor that the depth of self-revelation is not too great in early sessions. Initial self-disclosure is designed for group entry, not for major psychotherapeutic work. Powerful disclosure will shut down a group if there is not yet a base of confidence among the members. The therapist should be prepared to intervene when self-disclosure begins to escalate in the early sessions. The most effective way of doing this is to acknowledge the importance of the material with assurance that it will be dealt with in time. Comments such as, "I appreciate how difficult it is to talk about these very upsetting matters. It is good to introduce them now and we will certainly get back to explore them further with you later. I wonder if at the moment though we could pause and get some sense of reaction to what you have said or if other people have had similar types of experiences."

This problem of excessive disclosure may center around a group member who has a history of sabotaging the development of relationships by coming on too intensely or as too needy at an early point. This pattern may be replicated in the group, with the same result. One consistent finding in the group literature is that early self-disclosure is one of the predictors of premature termination. Dropouts often report that they were carried away in the enthusiasm of the early group and blurted out sensitive information. They may fear that they will be rejected or ridiculed, or that they have broken some personal or family taboo for which they will be blamed. This is one of the reasons for the value of the therapist having a personal meeting with a dropout. They may be in a critical state of decompensation and feel that there is no available help (40).

Completion of Stage 1

By the end of stage 1, group membership issues should be resolved. If the group is to lose members, it is usually done by this time.

There should be a general consensus of how the group operates as well as a reasonable sense of the group task. The therapist can consider the task of stage 1 to be nearing completion when all members are comfortable in participating and all have made some self-revealing statements indicating a basic trust in the group process.

For a weekly outpatient psychotherapy group, the first stage is usually accomplished in four to eight sessions. Some groups get off the ground more quickly than others, but a group that is still having difficulty with general positive participation after a couple of months is beginning to show developmental strains. When this emerges, the therapist needs to carefully review the group's life to that point, identifying the issues that seem to be interfering with progress and carefully considering strategies for addressing them.

It is important to understand that the first stage is not lacking in therapeutic effectiveness. It may be using the group process in a preliminary fashion, but the experience for the individual member can be powerful. The supportive factors that are mobilized address the demoralized state of many patients in a specific fashion. A positive shift in self-esteem results in a spiraling sense of self-confidence and self-efficacy that allows the individual to regain a sense of control. Once this is initiated, it may become a self-reinforcing process that allows continuing progress with or without the group.

Some groups stay in stage 1 work forever as a means for providing support for the members. Therapists who find themselves in settings in which it is necessary to keep reworking such issues should not become disillusioned with their task. Perhaps by conceptualizing it in terms of the specific dimensions outlined in this chapter, they can appreciate the importance of their work and understand how to maintain the appropriate focus without slipping inappropriately into interventions or expectations that are beyond the needs or capability of their patient population.

It is possible for groups to become stuck in stage 1. This may reflect the influence of a preponderance of members who fall on the sociable or structural role behavior spectrum. It may represent leadership difficulties about addressing issues of conflict or difference. Membership problems regarding attendance or terminations may thrust the group back to basic engagement tasks. Some groups leave the support and encouragement of early sessions, try to address more conflictual matters, retreat from these with a drop in cohesion, and then oscillate between the two stages. The material in this chapter and the next may offer some insights into how such a situation might be handled.

Summary

The engagement task of stage 1 focuses on the whole group. Individual issues are of less importance except as they threaten harm to the person, or obstruction to the group task. A modestly active therapeutic style is appropriate, particularly in reinforcing events falling into the support cluster of therapeutic factors. The mechanisms of stage 1 constitute an ongoing source of group cohesion. Therefore, they will come back into predominance any time that the work of the group is threatened. This regularly occurs at times of membership change or when difficult issues are being addressed.

Just as the positive developments of stage 1 are coming to fruition, the challenging tasks of stage 2 emerge. As a group moves through the engagement stage, the sense of group cohesion and commitment steadily increases. Once the stage tasks are achieved, the intensity may lessen, and a sense of vagueness or lack of direction may develop. The contributions of the divergent role members are often stimulated by this. The leader needs to be sensitive to an emerging sense of disillusionment or irritation. Once convinced that the group is together in mastering engagement tasks, the therapist can begin to promote the expression of more negative themes. Thus, the group can move on to stage 2, and we can move on to Chapter 9.

CHAPTER 9

Differentiation

The second stage of group development is called the differentiation stage. This stage is often referred to in the literature as the stage of conflict because it is characterized by an atmosphere of dissatisfaction and confrontation. The term *differentiation* focuses on the functional task of the stage for group development. The preoccupation with criticism and justification serves the purpose of developing a greater awareness of the individual in the group. This is a counterbalance to the assumptions of universality, uncritical acceptance, and similarities developed in stage 1. Although the work of stage 2 is not as pleasant as that of stage 1, it contributes greatly to the sense of groupness.

Basic Tasks

The central task for the group in stage 2 is to develop a cooperative approach to conflict resolution. This must begin with recognition by the group members that they do not all see the world the same way. The presence of different points of view threatens the sense of universality that initially allowed the members to get closer. Stage 2 focuses on the ability to tolerate differences and use them in a collaborative fashion.

Dealing With Conflict

Hints of the transition from stage 1 to stage 2 often center around minor complaints or dissatisfactions. Sometimes these are initially directed at issues outside of the group and then gradually come closer to issues within the group. Discontent with referral sources such as family doctors or with previous groups are common themes. Usually punctual members may appear late, and there are some unpredicted absences. There may be a mounting sense of frustration or irritation that is not directly addressed. There is an edgy confronting tone to the discussion, first between members and eventually toward the leader. A direct breakthrough of anger or criticism is a good sign that the work of the stage is progressing. In response to criticism, members make self-justifying assertions, often of an exaggerated nature. Several features of this group climate are specifically worth identifying.

Expression of negative affect.   Firmly, perhaps loudly stated opinions, challenges, criticisms, and misunderstandings may seem to contribute to an unproductive atmosphere. However, in this way the members become more self-disclosing, often by blurting out ideas or reactions that must then be defended. This process forces an increased appreciation of the uniqueness of each member and breaks down some of the unrealistic sense of commonality of stage 1. There is a great increase in the amount of information available about each individual. For these reasons, the members sense that the work is important, although not as enjoyable as it was in stage 1.

Identification of differences.   Opinions tend to be stated in terms of stereotypic descriptions that reflect a global judgment, not an individualized reaction. These should not be seen simply as the ventilation of negative affect but rather as statements of self-definition. It is typical of adolescents to see the world in polarized terms of good versus bad or acceptable versus unacceptable. This process promotes the development of a greater sense of autonomy and a clearer idea of self. The atmosphere during the differentiation stage of a group often has such an adolescent quality. The importance lies not so much in the actual content of the discussion, but in the process of self-assertion. By adopting this perspective, the therapist is able to intervene accurately by promoting and encouraging the exploration of differences among the members. This will defuse the affect constructively and permit the members to understand that they can continue to interact effectively even though they do not always agree.

Conflict resolution.   A further major task during this stage is the development of a group approach to conflict resolution. If this cannot be achieved, then the group becomes bottled up in unproductive criticism or self-justifying defensive rhetoric that may lead to a serious drop in group cohesion and member commitment. The approach to be fostered is one of exploring differences so that individual positions can be tolerated as neither right nor wrong, but rather different. Unresolvable competition can be replaced with a sense of cooperation, although not necessarily agreement.

The danger is that if this cognitive exploratory work does not take place, the group will either disintegrate or the tensions will go underground. The latter result may lead to a situation in which the group oscillates between the relatively superficial style of stage 1, punctuated by bursts of negative affect from repressed stage 2 material.

Leadership challenge.   Another feature that is central to the differentiation stage relates to the role of the therapist. Just as members identify differences between themselves, so the membership as a whole may identify differences between the group and the therapist. Criticism of the therapist frequently focuses on a perceived failure to care or provide enough: "You just get paid to do this and can't really know what we are experiencing," or "If you gave us more direction the group would be more helpful." This can be seen in one sense as the members needing to differentiate themselves from the "rules" laid down by the authorities. At a deeper level, it reflects disillusionment with the idea that the perfect solution is going to be provided by the therapist. During the engagement stage, the group was able to bask in the untested assumption that if everybody got along a healing process would occur without further work. It now appears that the process will be more challenging.

Reassessment of group norms.   The therapist's role in setting original group norms was clearly identified in preceding chapters. Now these ideas about how the group should operate must be critically examined. The importance of this process is that the members achieve a personal stake in how the group should function, resulting in an increased identification with, and sense of "ownership" of, the group. At the same time, the penetration and influence of the therapist is somewhat tempered. Underlying this process is a strengthening of normative expectations about the group. Usually, the results of this process are not greatly different from those at the beginning, but the process of challenging helps to make them more explicit. Here again there is a parallel to the necessary challenges of parental values and control that are characteristic of early adolescence.

There may be testing of group rules. Some members unconcernedly barge into sessions a few minutes late. There are whispered leaks about how the group assembled for coffee after the preceding session. These should be seen as minor transgressions in the service of a greater goal: the forging of a group consensus. For example, after several late arrivals, the group may have a serious discussion about how difficult it is to begin when members are late. Group pressure will be brought to bear on the tardy ones in a much more effective manner than possible from the therapist: "After all, it's *our* group now, not *yours*."

Dominance hierarchy.   Stage 2 phenomena may also be conceptualized as the enactment of the formation of a dominance hierarchy. This ranking process is part of our primate heritage. One of the first things to happen when a new group is formed is judgments about who has more influence. There is usually considerable agreement in the members' conclusions about this. Although these evaluations are initially made early in the group's life, in stage 2 they are tested. Much of the competitive jockeying at this time can be understood in this light (41).

The leadership challenge tests the top rung of the hierarchy—the therapist. One important way to describe a social system is the gradient of the dominance hierarchy. For example, in military groups it is absolutely prescribed. Therapy groups may vary considerably in the degree of therapist control. In general, greater member participation is achieved with a middle level of control. This reassures the members that someone is in a position of responsibility, but still accommodates member initiative. This idea is developed more completely in Chapter 12, where leader styles are described.

Boundary Focus

It will be clear from these descriptions that the boundary that now comes into focus is that of the individual member. In stage 1, it was important to identify information regarding differences between the group and outside experiences. Now it is important to focus on the public expression of internal information in the form of beliefs and reactions. Through this process, the individual begins to emerge as a more rounded and fully developed personality. Boundaries can be viewed as opening and closing. The typical stage 2 process of expression is the statement of a strongly held opinion followed by justification of that opinion. This represents a sequence of openness followed by closedness: an affect-driven self-disclosure followed by cognitive justification.

One particularly important example of the boundary focus is that between the therapist and the group members. On the group schematic presented in Chapter 3, the leadership subsystem boundary was identified. The work of stage 2 inevitably deals with issues across this boundary. Initially this may take the form of questions about leadership between a particular member or members and the leader. However, it commonly develops into a collective group stance about leadership that polarizes most of the group against the leader. This represents an illusion of unanimity in the service of the differentiation task. Given time and patience, the conflict resolution processes will allow the group to work through such issues.

Where Are the Therapeutic Factors?

It is important that the tasks of the differentiation stage be addressed on the foundation of solid group cohesion developed during the engagement stage. Groups that begin with high levels of conflict generally do not fare well because they do not have the positive cohesive "glue" to keep them together during the disintegrating effects of conflict resolution. It is for this reason that the therapist needs to dampen and divert conflictual themes in stage 1.

At first glance, it may appear that all those carefully nurtured supportive factors have disappeared. They are still very much present, but have now gone underground. Their presence is often leaked by the laugh and reconsolidation that occurs after a heated interchange. It is as if the members are saying, "We can get away with this heavy stuff, because we know we won't let each other down." The therapist may usefully remind the members from time to time that they do have a positive past together.

As mentioned above, the confrontational process results in further self-revelation. Indeed, the amount of personalized information available about each member often rises markedly through the second stage. The interactional process of stage 2 is laying the groundwork for the psychological work factors of insight and interpersonal learning in later stages.

Therapist Style and Technique

The general comments about therapist behavior in the preceding chapter continue to apply. The therapist should remain a predictable and sustaining force in the group. However, the change in group atmosphere does increase the pressure on the therapist. For the beginning therapist, it is useful to understand that stage 2 phenomena are basically constructive in nature. The process of therapist challenge is normal and inevitable. A defensive or apologetic response deprives the group of the opportunity to learn from the experience and may drive it back into an unsatisfying stage 1 condition. The following suggestions are intended to be superimposed on stage 1 techniques, not to replace them.

Keep calm.   The most important thing the therapist can do during this stage is to remain calm. This sends a powerful message to the members that nothing catastrophic is going to happen. It acknowledges the legitimacy of the issues, even if they are a bit overstated. The therapist needs to be careful not to intervene too soon in the group process, lest this be interpreted as an indirect message of concern, disapproval, or defensiveness.

There is a danger that the therapist may actively collude in the avoidance of the conflict of the differentiation stage. This may be based on the mistaken belief that the negative features may get out of hand or be destructive. If the therapist can tolerate stage 2 issues with equanimity, then the group has a chance to master them as well.

Explore differences.   The main technical task for the therapist in learning to manage this stage is to accurately label the central mechanism. This is not the expression of negative affect. A more powerful underlying mechanism is the exploration of different points of view. It is this dynamic that underlies the conflict and the sense of dissatisfaction characteristic of the stage.

The climate of stage 2 is typically characterized by the expression of polarized points of view. These may be expressed in an exaggerated tone of self-justification or outrage. They often entail a process of stereotyping people into less than desirable pigeonholes. This process is overdone, giving the impression of quite unrealistic assessments and perceptions. In the engagement stage, the uncritical acceptance of self-revelations in the service of universality and engagement occurred. Now, in stage 2, the process involves an unrealistic exaggeration of differences, still with a tendency to distortion. The process of confrontation increases the level of affect. This in turn results in pressure to disclose firmly held opinions or reveal negative and painful experiences. Such information may be blurted out in a burst of self-revelation. Once out, it must then be justified or defended, and this leads to some of the polarized and stereotypic statements. The need to defend one's position requires the revelation of strongly held beliefs or reactions that cut deeper into interpersonal issues. The result of this process is that the amount of personalized information available concerning each member is greatly expanded.

The therapist must develop a sense of timing regarding the point of optimum intervention. The affective climate should be allowed to reach a reasonable degree of intensity. This ensures that real interpersonal process tension is present. This feeling of an encounter makes the work productive. At an appropriate opportunity, the therapist can begin to shift the interchanges to a focus on the fact that members clearly are seeing things differently and encourage them to clarify their perception of the issues under discussion. This helps to validate each member's ideas and defines the process, not in terms of right or wrong, but in terms of varying viewpoints. The group can thus be led toward a mechanism for tension reduction based on cooperation. An optimum result is that the members can agree to disagree but continue working on the issues. This lays the base for greater tolerance in perceptions of others and the possibility of empathizing with people even in the face of disagreements. This will be very important for later group work. For example, as the group progresses, much discussion can be expected to center on misinterpretations concerning aspects of close relationships, including the contributions of various members. It is important that members can challenge such phenomena without their opinions being rejected outright. Stage 2 experiences lay the base for such work.

Manage leader challenge. During the first stage, the group operates under the guidelines laid down by the therapist in pretherapy preparation and the first few sessions. One of these normative expectations is that members should speak up about issues they are concerned about.

This idea of truthful openness about internal thoughts is central to all forms of therapy. It is somewhat of a paradox therefore that to obey this normative expectation means to challenge the very leader who stressed it in the first place.

The process of group challenge to the therapist plays an important part in the work of this stage. It reveals a deeper commitment by the individual to the group process and a higher investment in the resulting normative shift. Not surprisingly, this process often has a somewhat adolescent quality to it. It is as if the members know that some of the issues they are raising are of less than central importance, yet they are bound to vigorously make their points. Just as adolescents establish close peer relationships, so the group during this phase bands together as a group of "co-rebels" determined to alter the system. There is minimal danger that nontherapeutic norms will eventually prevail. What is critical is that a leader has been challenged and everyone has survived.

The response of the leader to the challenging process will help or hinder the mastery of the stage tasks. The therapist must not respond with an intensification of rules or authoritarian or judgmental statements. Nor should the issues be trivialized by ignoring them or shutting down discussions of them. A few deep breaths to recognize the inevitability of the process are useful, and a parental perspective of "this too shall pass" is a great asset. If the group believes that therapist challenge is not permissible or not safe, it may revert back to the safety of stage 1 or may seek an alternative outlet by identifying a group member as a scapegoat to receive the negative attitudes deflected from the leader.

Address the fear of the individual. A common fear of members as they engage in stage 2 work is that the interpersonal challenges will be destructive. This may take the form of concern that other members will not be able to tolerate criticism and may be driven from the group. An associated fear is that oneself will be found unacceptable for uttering critical or angry words. Fears such as these will be universally present. It is useful therefore for the therapist to put them into words and to review with the members how they are reacting to the process. In most cases, members are able to say that they may not be comfortable with the process but can manage. Some groups come to an agreement that members can call for a "time-out" if they find themselves having difficulty mastering the process.

Prevent harmful interactions. The therapist must be alert to over-powering messages of blame or rejection between members that may prove damaging. It is useful to check members' reactions to group events to forestall this. The therapist has a clear responsibility to monitor the confrontational process and to ensure that no one is harmed and must be prepared to intervene if that appears to be a danger. Techniques for this are discussed below in the section on scapegoating (42).

The Individual Member

A challenge for the individual member during the second stage is to tolerate a negative group atmosphere with its dimensions of hostility, conflict, and confrontation. Patients presenting for psychotherapy often have difficulty in either over- or underexpression of anger. Therefore, the work of stage 2 is generally relevant to many members. The therapist needs to monitor carefully that this is proceeding in a constructive fashion and that the affective issues are being mastered through the cognitive mechanisms described above.

The individual must arrive at a comfortable position regarding acceptance of social norms versus continuing in a challenging position during stage 2. Although part of the group task is to throw the question of normative expectations up in the air, the resolution is to come down with a general agreement concerning them. Thus, it is to be expected that members who are strong on the divergent role will come out of this period with their need to challenge authority under some-what greater cognitive control. They will be able to use this constructive quality in a functional, not a dysfunctional, fashion. This may be a central therapeutic accomplishment for such individuals.

While the group challenging is going on, a parallel process is found within the individual. Just as individual members are challenged within the group, so components of self-image and self-perceptions are also raised for consideration. Material tentatively raised in stage 1 must come under greater scrutiny. During the differentiation stage, the individual is more likely to become aware of parts of self that are in an uneasy alliance or are frankly contradictory. Split-off or isolated interpersonal fragments may come to the fore. These may be the source of intense reactions of guilt and shame. The general sense of anxiety, confrontation, and disgruntlement in the air may be seen in part as a projection from these internal dimensions.

The therapist needs to look for evidence of such introspective work and encourage exploration of these themes. Questions such as, "It seems as if you can behave in two different ways with different people. With your mother you seem to be always obedient and accepting, whereas with your wife you need to find fault with everything she does." The therapist has a powerful tool available in identifying parallel processes going on within the individual and within the group. The group application functions rather like a projection of internal issues onto the persons in the group. What is difficult to discern in the smaller image of the person becomes evident when it is projected onto the larger screen of the group.

The pressure during this stage to justify and defend oneself provides an informal experience in assertiveness training. Indeed, the therapist may want to incorporate some aspects of this modality into the management technique. An important by-product of this process is the opportunity to create a more complex self-definition. This builds on the focus on self as an object of concern that characterized stage 1.

Social Roles

The social role most in focus during the differentiation stage is the divergent role, the scapegoat in the group. It will be clear from the description of the divergent role behaviors that their emergence will be promoted during stage 2. These members eagerly express contrary viewpoints. They are intuitively aware of process events, particularly that aspect of process dealing with evasive or defensive behavior. They are ready to dive in and identify avoidant behaviors and label the issues. This is often done in a blunt and relatively tactless fashion.

With these activities, the divergent role members are contributing a vital ingredient to the task of addressing stage 2 issues. Groups without such members will experience difficulty in coming to terms with conflictual themes. Therapists must learn to value and acknowledge their divergent scapegoats. Without them, the task will be much harder. The therapist must be careful not to align with the other members in attacking the scapegoat. These people often lay themselves open for abuse and seem to relish the process even though they may be hurting inside. Their vigorous and extroverted methods may obscure the pain they experience at perceiving themselves once again on the outside. The therapist may need to offer support to the scapegoat not only in terms of role behavior but also in regard to self-esteem. This can be done through acknowledging the contribution that person is making to the work of the group. It can also be rein-forced by acknowledging the validity of the issues being raised.

During stage 2, the functions of the sociable and structural role leaders continue to be important. They are the culture bearers of cohesive engagement. The sociable role members in particular will be appalled to see their "nice group" apparently unraveling around them. They will need some reassurance that group cohesion will be able to survive the confrontational process. Structural role members are more comfortable bridging the changing climate because of the stress they place on task accomplishment. They also represent the autonomy axis and can understand the importance of individual perceptions and opinions. They are helpful in working through differentiation issues.

The cautionary role members, who have come to a grudging acceptance of the group system in stage 1, will find in the tumult of stage 2 the confirmation of their worst fears about group participation. Attention will be required from the therapist to ensure that their motivation continues. They may be able to offer constructive thoughts about the importance of the individual. Such comments may be presented in an angry or critical manner that aligns these members with those in the divergent role position.

Predictable Problems

Projective Mechanisms

During stage 2, projective defense mechanisms are in evidence. *Projection* refers to the unconscious attribution of thoughts or feelings that are one's own to another person. This is understood as a way of managing self-evaluations that are considered unacceptable or dan-gerous. Such phenomena are a regular feature of psychotherapy groups, more so than in individual therapy, making groups a particu-larly advantageous place to observe projective mechanisms at work. Generally, the group phenomena of displacement and projection onto a given member can be handled through an exploration of the differ-ences in viewpoint as discussed earlier in this chapter (43).

Projective Identification

The use of projective identification leads to serious distortions in interpersonal perceptions. It is based on a situation in which internal perceptions of the self as both good and bad exist in separate compartments. The individual may fluctuate from one state to another, seeing himself or herself as special and entitled at one time and as evil and destructive at others. These internal perspectives are then projected onto separate people. This results in a splitting process so that some group members come to be viewed in unrealistically positive terms, whereas others are viewed in totally negative terms. If stress develops in one of these relationships, there may be a sudden shift from positive to negative.

This more extreme form of the projection mechanism is seen particularly in patients with difficulties in basic object relations as described in borderline personality disorders. Such patients have difficulty in clearly defining themselves, and they tend to fuse their perception of self into that of the other. Therefore, both positive and negative relationships become highly charged. The individual behaves toward the other person as if he or she possesses the projected characteristics. This often elicits from the other the very behaviors they are anticipating, which confirms and consolidates the projective identification process. Patients with this tendency are likely to use any movement toward group scapegoating as a vehicle for an extension of their personal projections. They may lead the group in this direction and carry it beyond levels at which it can be easily addressed. The intensity of psychopathology of such patients makes it difficult for them to utilize cognitive meditating mechanisms. It is for this reason that caution needs to be taken in placing such patients in a group therapy situation in which the social milieu will tend to inflame their distorting propensities. The use of homogeneous groups for patients with borderline personality features may be considered. These groups can move at a slower pace with careful and systematic attention to the distorting mechanisms.

The Scapegoat

The metaphor of the scapegoat originates in the Old Testament, as part of the ritual associated with the annual Day of Atonement:

And Aaron shall lay both his hands upon the head of the live goat, and confess over him all the inequities of the children of Israel, and all their transgressions in all their sins, putting them upon the head of the goat, and shall send him away by the hand of a fit man into the wilderness: And the goat shall bear upon him all their inequities unto a land not inhabited: and he shall let go the goat in the wilderness. (The Holy Bible [Authorized Version] Leviticus 16:21-22)

The designation of a scapegoat demonstrates the projective mechanism at work in the social system. A group consensus forms that if a particular member were no longer in the group, everyone else could get along satisfactorily. This allows the other group members to become unified and still deal with themes involving negative affect. This displacement process can be seen as a group mechanism for dealing with the conflict inherent in the differentiation work. It represents an unstable compromise because the collaborating members are at the same time denying that other differences exist among them. If the chosen scapegoat leaves the group, then the process must be repeated in order to maintain the defensive position. Groups may go through several members in this fashion.

A variant on this process is for the group to agree on an external source of the problem. This may be a collective agreement that men are the problem in a group of women, or that the school system is the problem in a group of parents. This group-level mechanism is a reflection in the collectivity of the group of the same sort of projective process as may occur in the individual. It is the phenomenon Bion described in basic assumption fight/flight states.

The therapist must be ready to intervene if the scapegoating process becomes overly active. Patients who become group casualties report being the victim of this process and suffering humiliation and severe damage to their self-esteem. The therapist has several possible approaches to consider.

Identify the source of conflict.   The presence of a scapegoating pattern reflects some underlying issue with which the group is trying to grapple. If this can be identified and dealt with, then the need for a scapegoat vanishes. Often the real target is the therapist, who may have been giving mixed messages about the acceptability of leader challenges.

Support the scapegoat.   Others in the group may share some of the opinions being promoted by the identified scapegoat. If these members can join the scapegoat then there is less danger. The therapist may need to align himself with the scapegoat. This is done most smoothly at an early point in the process: "I hear everybody getting on Jim's back about these things, but it seems to me that he has a valid point." Sometimes simply letting the scapegoat know that his or her role is being appreciated provides enough support.

Halt the process.   When all else fails, the therapist may need to specifically call a halt to the process: "I think this has gone on long enough and everybody has things out of perspective. Let's put the subject on hold for tonight and see how it looks next week." This, by the way, is a well-recognized function of a primate alpha male. He functions as a referee to ensure that the process of displaced aggression between high-ranking animals does not go too far.

Completion of Stage 2

The successful outcome of stage 2 entails an undertaking to cooperate, not necessarily to agree, as was the case in stage 1. Failure to master this process has one of two predictable outcomes: 1) The group may grind on in a chronically dissatisfied competitive fashion with ebbing morale and gradual loss of members. 2) The group may bounce back into the less critical atmosphere of stage 1. This will soon become boring or dissatisfying so that the group will likely keep testing conflictual issues only to rebound each time. This may continue for extended periods of time, the therapist recognizing that something is not working but not quite able to identify the problem.

It is common for stage 2 to build in intensity and then rather suddenly settle. The therapist may leave one session wondering where the group is headed, only to begin the next with a group settled into a determined stance of collaborative work. As in all stages, it is important that each member participates in the work of the stage.

Summary

The differentiation stage contributes to the normative development of the group. Through the process of leader challenge, the group gains a more consolidated view of its nature and functions. In this process, individual members become more recognizable in terms of greater information and interactional activity. The therapist carries a responsibility to ensure that no member is hurt by the negative atmosphere.

Stages 1 and 2 are sometimes referred to as *prework* stages. They lay the groundwork for more complex interpersonal functioning and the capacity for more sensitive levels of empathy. Groups that have mastered these tasks are equipped to be engaged and supporting while at the same time able to deal with differences and confrontation.

It is important to bear in mind that useful therapeutic work may occur during these two early stages. They represent interaction focused on the two major diagonal axes of the Structural Analysis of Social Behavior interpersonal space, anchored in the trust/support quadrant for stage 1, and the blame/protest quadrant for stage 2. In many situations, circumstances preclude groups from moving beyond early-stage phenomena. Therapists in such groups should not despair that they are never really getting to do group therapy. Good work during stages 1 and 2 is often all that many patients require to initiate a personal change process.

The Later Group

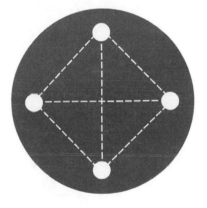

CHAPTER **10**

The Working Group

The term *working group* is used in a special way. In the discussion concerning group composition, it was suggested that groups be ranked in terms of the degree to which interpersonal learning would constitute an important part of the experience. Although interpersonal learning takes place in all groups, it is useful to consider how central it will be for therapist strategy. In the engagement and differentiation stages, most therapist attention is directed toward facilitating the formation of a therapeutic milieu. Individual issues are used to promote group growth but are not the principal focus. Once the tasks of the early group are accomplished, more emphasis can be directed at the learning to be gained from understanding the personal implications of the relationships that are forming between group members. It is from this perspective that the first two stages can be considered *prework* stages, and those following as *working* stages (44).

There is considerable therapeutic potential in the engagement and differentiation stages. These stages may be quite a profound experience for the individual member and may set off a series of changes in attitudes or behavior that begin an ongoing constructive process. In this sense, the individual members are "working" from the very beginning. However, from the standpoint of the group system, a more predictable interactional climate that focuses on psychological change emerges at a later point. The group has learned by this time that there are similarities between the members so they can understand each other and also that they can disagree and confront each other. This gives the group greater ability to focus on, and work through, resistances and differences of opinion. A greater openness for self-revelation, a receptivity to feedback from others, and an introspective attitude that can incorporate such feedback is required for this. By conceptualizing the time-limited group in developmental terms, the therapist can specifically work to accelerate progress through stages 1 and 2 so that more time is available for the working stages.

Advanced Developmental Stages

The process of the group interaction has many common features during the three working stages of individuation, intimacy, and mutuality. Progress is revealed by a series of shifts in content themes and relationship focus. There is greater overlap between these stages than in the more discrete content of the engagement and differentiation stages. Nonetheless, recognition of the underlying central concern of each stage can direct the therapist toward well-targeted interventions. To use a musical analogy, it is as if the key signature changes. The melody line may still be there, but the shift from a major to a minor key lends it a different significance.

Individuation Stage

The individuation stage is characterized by a focus on introspective work. Although this takes place through an interactive process, the content deals with understanding the individual in more depth. The shift into this work from the active interactions of stage 2 results in a decrease in tension in the group. The introspective process not only increases the understanding the members have of each other, but also decreases interpersonal resistance to psychological exploration. The ability to confront in a collaborative fashion is now put to constructive use. This process results in an appreciation of the complexity of the self and the beginning recognition of conflictual issues as they arise in relationships. In this stage, much material relating to the family of origin emerges. These memories may "turn on" old response patterns that influence group relationships. These will form an important focus for group learning.

This idea of "turning on" old patterns is another way of describing regression. The introspective process takes the individual back in memory to earlier relationship situations. Behavior characteristic of those times is then incorporated into here-and-now group interaction, creating a state of isomorphy between developmental patterns and group events. Thus, by focusing on present group events, the therapist is at the same time addressing early learned patterns regarding relationships and self-concept.

Intimacy Stage

As a result of the introspective focus, the members learn a great deal about each other. This information draws them closer together and leads to the work focus of the intimacy stage. The therapist may want to hold the group in the introspective process until it is clear that all members have participated in such work. Increasing knowledge about each other inevitably leads to greater commitment to therapeutic work between members.

The thematic shift to intimacy stage material may emerge first through detailed exploration of outside intimate relationships. This moves the group from introspective material back to an interpersonal agenda. For many patients, this is both an attraction and a danger. If previous close relationships have ended in experiences of loss or harm, the prospect of new closeness may be very threatening. Some members may experience a fear that the intensity of the group may overwhelm them.

The opportunity to explore the implications of closeness can flourish more actively in groups than in individual therapy where role disparity has a tempering effect. There is a danger that the group will come to replace real-life relationships. This may lead to a withdrawal from outside personal relationships that do not seem to have the intensity and the safety of those found within the group. Questions of romantic feelings between members must be explored openly so that unrealistic expectations or distorted fears can be understood. This possibility is discussed in more detail later in this chapter.

Mutuality Stage

The exploration of intimacy leads to a consideration of the responsibilities of closeness. Members must face not only the pleasures of relationships but also the frustrations and disappointments that may accompany them. This activates issues related to individual autonomy versus interdependence. At one extreme, an excessive need for autonomy may lead to isolation and avoidance of relationships. At the other, enmeshment in a relationship may preclude individual decisions.

Greater interdependence brings with it the need to resolve a power dimension of control/exploitation versus submission. Members may experience a fear of vulnerability and of becoming trapped in a relationship of unequal status. To address this fear, they must be prepared to place appropriate demands on others and to judiciously limit the commitments they make. The question of personal responsibility brings the group to a mature level of functioning that often involves existential themes of self-identity and meaning.

Movement of Group Work

The movement of the group through the sequence of stage tasks allows each member to work through issues related to the principal dimensions of interpersonal functioning. As in individual growth and development, there is a certain quality of repetition involved as if spiraling to deeper levels of understanding. The engagement stage deals with affiliation themes that emerge again at a more personal level in the intimacy stage. The differentiation stage involves issues of power and control that reappear in the mutuality stage. The individuation stage, serving as a retreat inward, provides greater information and trust that enables the members to begin to address deeper levels of the spiral.

Table 10-1 lists the characteristics of each stage. This table may be used in conjunction with Figure 5-1 as a map for plotting the movement of group work. The process of therapy may be conceptualized as one in which these phenomena are opened more or less sequentially for discussion by the group. By "massaging" the stage-appropriate concepts, the members will be drawn in the direction of productive therapeutic work. This is managed by relatively simple techniques that indicate an interest in, and the need for clarification about, the thematic material in question.

For example, in the intimacy stage, discussion about outside relationships may first be expanded by encouraging a discussion about the meaning the events held for the individual. This often brings out issues of self-esteem, acceptance, support, and perhaps disillusionment. Once this information about the interpersonal meaning of intimate relationships is available, the therapist can wonder what it is like to talk about such personal matters in the group: "Who seems to

Table 10-1. Stage developmental model

Stage	Boundary focus	Group task	Threat to individual	Mechanism to resolve threat	Individual task—attendant danger	Index to task resolution
Engagement	External group	Develop group identity and cohesion	Unacceptability	Universality; preliminary self-revelation	"We're all the same" (untested universality)	Acceptance of membership; commitment to participate
Differentiation	Individual member	Develop mechanism of conflict resolution through cooperative exploration	Conflict	Cooperative exploration; assertion of ideas and beliefs	"I'm somewhat different" (unrealistic polarizations)	Tolerance of difference; conflict resolution
Individuation	Intrapsychic	Develop understanding of individual through self-revelation and reflective introspection	Loss of self-esteem	Reflective introspection; deeper self-revelation	"I'm a complex but whole person" (morbid self-preoccupation)	Acceptance of self and others; collaborative exploration
Intimacy	Intermember	Develop interpersonal involvement and allow reciprocal influence	Rejection	Reciprocal influence; acknowledging importance of relationships	"I can be important to someone else" (irresponsible closeness)	Tolerance of closeness; nondefensive openness
Mutuality	Intermember	Develop understanding of equality in relationships, not dependence/exploitation	Inequality	Quality in relationships; accepting implications of one's actions for others	"What I do has implications for someone else" (unrealistic closeness)	Acceptance of personal responsibility in relationships; management of dominance/control
Termination	External group	Allow individual autonomy and incorporate group experience	Aloneness	Incorporation of group; acknowledging loss	"I can exist even though alone" (nihilism)	Acceptance of responsibility for self; review and acknowledgment of group's importance

Source. Reprinted with permission from Dies and MacKenzie 1983. Copyright 1983 International Universities Press.

understand you best in here?" " What was your reaction to that pretty intense exchange you two had earlier about your respective spouses?" "Was it frightening as well as satisfying (exciting? comforting?) to go through that?" "Can you tell him what it meant to you to hear that?" This probing of both outside and in-group relationships permits comparisons to be drawn that illuminate the group events, while encouraging application to outside situations.

These stages will appear naturally in groups. In the best of circumstances, the therapist can follow the progressive development of this thematic material, gently reinforcing the process. When resistances appear, a more vigorous approach to clarify the issues is required. The progression through stage tasks may not always be in a forward direction. It is to be expected that any change in group membership, for example, will force the group to rework engagement issues, generally more quickly than the first time around. When the group is dealing with issues that are of particular difficulty for many of the members, then regressive behavior may emerge. Bion's ideas of "basic assumption" states of dependency and fight/flight may be seen as alternative ways of describing regression to stages 1 and 2, respectively. By the nature of their goals, some groups are expected to stay in early engagement work. In these, the therapist may actively resist group efforts to move on into conflictual material.

The developmental stage perspective gives the therapist a vantage point for assessing the general nature of group interaction and thus a base from which to make knowledgeable decisions regarding the need for interventions.

Interpersonal Learning

Interpersonal learning forms the basic rationale for group psychotherapy. Such learning is also implied in the corrective emotional experience of individual psychotherapy (45). In the group context, the nature of the learning process is rather different. The peer interaction of a group does not entail the influence and power of the professional role. Instead, it offers the reality of interacting with people who are experiencing the same sort of problems. This gives the interchanges a quality of genuineness that adds to the therapeutic effect. One of the major strengths of therapy in a group is the manner in which group members can get at important issues or penetrate defensive style because they are peers. Insightful comments from another group member cannot be easily dismissed as coming from someone who "doesn't understand my situation" or discounted as not applying to the realities of life outside the group.

Problems may arise for therapists who consider the main therapeutic impact to reside primarily in their own efforts. They are liable to interfere with the therapeutic power available from the group system. Frequent use of interpretive statements to individual members will move the group into a leader-oriented style in which each member strives to find "the answer" from the leader. Instead, a major function of the therapist is to constantly promote therapeutic events between the members, a field of action that offers infinitely more variability. The therapist must have faith in the resources of understanding available within the group membership. By fostering member-to-member interaction, the therapist is enhancing the opportunity of members to help each other and to have practice in applying new psychological learning in a real social situation.

Therapist activity is appropriately used to ensure that the group stays focused on its task. This may involve bringing the group back to reconsider a statement just made. It may mean probing for further reactions or eliciting responses from a greater number of group members. The therapist may be able to compare and contrast between some of the responses, thus revealing important differences in how members react to the same events. The overall result is an intensification of the group interactive process. This may be described as promoting the here-and-now process by stimulating action over a diversity of boundaries. A group that has developed therapeutic interactional norms will be able to carry much of the work of interpersonal learning with some assistance from the therapist. It is therapeutic for the members to experience a greater sense of self-responsibility for maintaining the working atmosphere.

In the following material in this section, it may seem that the mechanisms of interpersonal learning are discussed primarily in cognitive terms. It must be kept in mind that for the patient, this is an absorbing and powerful process. The therapist can deepen the experience by exploring the emotional reactions of the participants. Typical questions might be, "What was it like to speak of these matters that you have always kept secret?" "The experience of telling him what you disliked about his answer sounds like you took a risk in the group; how was it?" "What sort of reactions are getting stirred up by their comments to you?"

Intense emotional expression is only a part of the total corrective emotional experience. It is not an end in itself. Indeed, members who have critical experiences that are solely emotional tend to have less satisfactory outcomes. Integration of the meaning of the experience through cognitive understanding assists the process of internalization and application. It also serves to bind the affective component to specific issues rather than having it spread inappropriately over all situations. For example, it is one thing to be mad at all men, another to be mad at all controlling men, and different still to be mad at a specific controlling man. The exploration of affect is only the starting point. Once the affect is mobilized, an understanding of its meaning provides an opportunity for applied learning (46).

The Johari Window

In Chapter 7 (see Appendix), a diagram was used in the pretherapy preparation material as a way of conceptualizing how learning can occur in a group. This diagram is called the Johari Window (47). In a simple fashion, it encapsulates the idea of psychological processes that may interfere with interpersonal functioning. It recognizes the existence of material hidden either purposefully or because it is not available to the individual through unconscious mechanisms. It acknowledges the importance of learning from things others tell you about yourself, as well as from an introspective process. The format of the Johari Window is easily grasped by patients and can be used as a rationale for the psychotherapeutic learning cycle.

The Johari format can also guide the therapist in tracking group process. The goal of therapy may, in one sense, be to increase the amount of "public knowledge." This may be accomplished through self-disclosures by the patient, through which information is transferred from the "hidden" box to the "public" box. Similarly, feedback to the individual from others transfers information known to others into the public box where it is understood by the patient as well. The process of personal insight is reflected in movement across the "known/unknown to self" boundary. In practice, all of these events may be going on simultaneously. However, by considering them as specific components of the learning situation, the therapist can identify and reinforce them. This provides another boundary-managing technique.

In Chapter 2, a somewhat similar two-by-two matrix (Figure 2-1) was used to consider group norms. In that context also the goal was to increase behaviors under positive normative control by encouraging "risky" behaviors and having them validated. Norms are the social system equivalent to personal criteria regarding appropriate behavior and they reflect internal values or fears. Such attitudes take their shape from early experiences. As the group strives to clarify the relationships among the members, the members must apply the issues raised to their own situation. These ideas of the Johari Window and of the norm matrix provide parallel information structures.

Self-disclosure

This mechanism moves information from the category of "personal secrets" to that of "public knowledge." In early group sessions, self-disclosure tends to be mainly factual and increases in levels of personal sensitivity with time. At a pragmatic level, it is obvious that people must say something about themselves if they are to address personal problems.

The personal secrets box has some interesting implications. The withholding of information is a component of interpersonal deceit. This is a perfectly normal process. We choose to tell things about ourselves when we judge the situation to be safe. To tell too little is to be interpersonally overly cautious. To tell too much is to be interpersonally naive. Self-disclosure therefore has a direct relationship to levels of trust and, in groups, cohesion. This is one reason so much emphasis has been put on preparing patients for groups. By facilitating a rapid sense of groupness, the therapist is at the same time creating the conditions for increased self-disclosure.

As the group develops, it is to be expected that the nature of self-disclosure will shift into more introspective areas of personal feelings and also into interactional areas of giving feedback to others by revealing reactions to what others say. In addition, if the therapeutic process is advancing satisfactorily, the individual member will begin to have access to some material from the unknown area. An emerging sense of internal conflicts or contradictory and split-off parts within the self may pose critical decisions about self-disclosure. Often this sort of material is accompanied by deep feelings of shame or incompetence. It may involve behaviors that have been kept hidden, or feelings and reactions about significant others that have never been shared. To acknowledge these publicly to the group may have a powerful therapeutic effect. To keep them hidden may lead to disengagement. The therapeutic factor of catharsis lends much of the power to this experience.

The therapist must pay close attention to the interactional process at times of significant new self-revelations. In some way, a group response to the material should be engineered. It can be a painful experience to reveal long-hidden experiences or reactions and get no response at all. It is also important to check on how the revealing member has tolerated the group process. Because secrets are often associated with strong affect, the member may misunderstand or misinterpret what others say in response. By debriefing the episode before the session ends, the therapist can be sure that the experience was not a negative one. In addition, a review of the process will begin to desensitize the revealed material and thus facilitate cognitive mastery over it.

Interpersonal Feedback

Interpersonal feedback is a complementary mechanism to self-disclosure. It provides the individual with information about the impact of his or her behavior on others. If received and acknowledged, this may stimulate an introspective process. Feedback may, for example, involve a supportive or understanding reaction to some quality in, or information about, the other. It may identify a discrepancy between nonverbal behavior and verbal content. It often involves alternative viewpoints about perspectives or attitudes. In general, it enhances the ability to understand the real effect one has on others.

The group context offers some advantages over individual therapy in this regard. Interpretive or confrontational messages are frequently more easily accepted from other group members than from the therapist. This may be related to the dimension of control or power, making it easier to accept such statements from one's peers than from the leader. At the same time, the members offering such statements are participating in an altruistic process of helping others. Others members may benefit vicariously by watching and thinking about the exchanges. A well-developed working atmosphere can be a potent vehicle for introspective work.

The process of feedback has a theoretical base in operant conditioning. Positive feedback is that which increases the targeted behavior. Negative feedback is that which decreases it. Most systems operate primarily on the principles of negative feedback. In the group psychotherapy setting, both positive and negative feedback loops may be desirable. For example, for the withdrawn patient who has difficulty in assertion and self-presentation, positive feedback of encouragement and support may be effective in increasing these behaviors. For a person with impulse control difficulties, negative feedback is appropriate to decrease such episodes.

Now we come to the difficulties. *Positive* and *negative* as used above do not necessarily imply positive and negative emotional tone. For example, a strong reaction of anger or criticism to an impulsive gesture may actually provide positive reinforcement for it. One of the technical challenges of working in groups is how to effectively set limits and provide corrective negative feedback. Simple lack of response or diversion to another topic is a common negative feedback technique. But, in general, learning is augmented when the process is more explicit. Several guidelines are available for maximizing the use of feedback. These are simple mechanisms, at first glance seemingly beneath the dignity of a graduated professional, but they are frequently ignored. By attending to these principles, the infrastructure of the change induction process can be carefully constructed (48).

1. *Begin with the positive.*   This establishes a receptive atmosphere that promotes a collaborative response. Search for positive features of the situation that can be reinforced, evidence of some strength or determination. The idea is to support the individual even though dealing with excessive or dysfunctional behavior. This avoids an implied condemnation of the whole person.
2. *Identify the target.*   This best follows a positive aligning comment. This sequence can increase motivation for change while providing specific information about what to work on. The focus may be on overt behavior or internal thought processes.
3. *Be rational.*   The therapist is in a position to model an approach that emphasizes understanding before judgment. In particular, a strong expression of therapist anger or criticism reflects a loss of the "therapeutic attitude" of aligning with the patient against problematic behaviors. It is also one of the commonly cited reasons for negative effects.
4. *Be consistent.*   Once a particular issue has been identified, do not let it disappear. At the same time, reinforce changes in adaptation. Often, therapeutic effect is seen first in subtle shifts in behavior that reflect a reordering of internal priorities or attitudes.
5. *Use the group.*   The goal is to train the group members to be of help to each other. The impact of feedback is greater if all members can apply it with skill.

Feedback is a technical term that may be misused in its therapeutic application. In fact, it might be suggested that therapists not even use the word *feedback* in clinical work. Nine times out of ten it invokes an image of "now it's our turn to get him," and feedback time turns into verbal flagellation. It is easy for the therapist who is experienced in the process of therapy to forget just how important comments from the leader or members can be. One major advantage of group therapy is the power of the group to induce change. This same power can be destructive. The therapist must assume responsibility for monitoring the nature of this loop and actively intervene to modulate negative criticism. In particular, any evidence of a malicious intent to harm or reject must be addressed promptly.

Strongly expressed negative criticism is commonly fueled by the personal issues of the person delivering it. Exploration of both sides of the process is therefore warranted. The therapist may need to provide support to the recipient, not necessarily by denying or dismissing the issues being raised, but by assisting in the ability to use such information. Introspective work may carry with it a threat to the individual's sense of self-esteem. The support derived from a cohesive group environment usually addresses this adequately, but the therapist should keep a watchful eye that the individual member can tolerate the process. Feedback, from both the therapist and the members, is most effective if it originates from the therapeutic attitude that is directed at aspects of the person's behavior, not the whole person.

The learning cycle of self-disclosure and interpersonal feedback may move in both directions. Self-disclosure will stimulate responses from others, and feedback may trigger self-disclosure. Both mechanisms result in a clarification of issues about the individual and about the impact that the individual makes on others. These basic processes are at the heart of therapeutic change.

Introspection

It is the nature of introspective work that it deals with material that is hidden to the individual, is highly charged with affect, and may involve significant distortions in how the individual sees the interpersonal world. The therapist can assist the group in introspective work by continually translating material of an intrapsychic nature into its interpersonal application. For example, if a patient is experiencing guilt, it might be useful to find out who in the group the patient feels has the most critical attitude toward his or her story or behavior. By using such techniques, the therapist can promote the enactment of the interpersonal behavior, which will demonstrate and open up important issues.

Because of the opportunity in groups for many different types of relationships to emerge, a broad panorama is available on which the individual can display the types of relationships that are both adaptive or problematic. To put this in formal language, there is the opportunity for multiple transferences to occur within a group in a manner that is quite different from that in individual therapy. The introspective process can be accelerated by utilizing these various relationships to focus on those that are more functional and contrast these with others that reveal dysfunction.

The therapist can expedite the learning process with the systematic use of clarification—clarification about what the individual knows about self and what can be expressed to others; clarification about what others find in each individual's presentation and can clarify back. Whenever a member makes a personally important statement, the primary task of the therapist is not to offer interpretations but rather to elicit the response of other group members. Usually these produce a rich network of reactions and ideas, often of a quite sophisticated nature.

Another way of describing the process of interpersonal learning is through the language of personal construct theory (49), which focuses on the manner in which individuals construe their interpersonal world. For example, the depressed person systematically picks out the most negative interpretations to apply to current events, the past, and the future. At a more complex level, these "personal construct" ideas may be applied to an understanding of the dimensions used by people to explain their relationships. An idiosyncratic view of the interpersonal world is actively manufactured through the application of unique sets of ideas about people. This has been described as an attempt to provide a sense of regularity to one's experiences. Kelly (1955) defined a psychological disorder as a "personal construction that is used repeatedly in spite of consistent invalidation." For example, a common pattern in neurotic men is a strong link between the constructs of love and weakness. Thus the idea of being in an intimate relationship automatically calls up an association with being weak and passive. This personal construct orientation is relevant to the idea of defining a characteristic theme of interpersonal tension as the focus for therapeutic attention.

Critical Incidents

One way of organizing and conceptualizing group events is to consider a session as a series of critical incidents. This orientation is useful at any point in a group's life. It is described in detail here because the focus on specific learning episodes is particularly important once the group is equipped for more challenging work. Not only can critical incidents be used to track group events as they occur, such episodes are also useful in reporting groups for purposes of supervision (50).

The idea of critical incidents is only one way of considering group interactions, one selection from a continuum of time frames. Sometimes it is useful to think of the entire group experience, from start to finish, as a unit. This might be useful in comparing the features of a group for anorexic patients and a group for schizophrenic patients. Another perspective already used in this book is to consider the group in terms of a series of developmental stages, each lasting a number of sessions. A tighter time frame is to view each full session as a unit. This is reflected in studies using group climate reports in which the members are asked to describe the group as a whole during a single session. Critical incidents, our concern in this section, divide the action up into segments lasting a number of minutes. Many research studies using videotape or transcript analysis focus on even shorter time segments, a single utterance as the unit of attention. Each of these time frames has its own value and focuses on different aspects of groupness.

The idea of a critical incident has some similarity to the use of short interpersonal stories to complete a relationship theme, the Core Conflictual Relationship Theme (CCRT), to use Luborsky's semistructured interview as described in Chapter 6. Within any given group session there might be several such events. If this number grows beyond 10 or 12, the therapist should use less detail and look for larger thematic segments.

A critical incident is defined as having a common theme, a common emotional tone, and often a subset of active group members involved in it. It is sometimes possible to identify the specific action that initiated the critical incident and then to track the swell of attention around that particular focus as it crests and then begins to wind down. Good therapists probably think this way intuitively. They are able to align with the current thematic material at an early point and thus reinforce its presence. They then sense when that theme is beginning to lose its intensity and the time is ripe for "processing" it. A critical learning event has been described as characterized by elevated affect, an attempt at new and risky behavior, a realization that the feared catastrophic result did not occur, and finally an opportunity to work through the entire situation from a reality orientation (51).

A critical incident is a useful time unit for the therapist to use in applying many of the ideas in this book. Each incident can be viewed from many perspectives.

Group structure.   An incident can be scanned in terms of a group structural diagram, focusing in turn on each boundary and considering the three levels of the system hierarchy: the group system, interactions between members, and internal issues. What boundary focus best captures the essence of the process? An involvement boundary can be drawn around the key participants. Would it be useful to compare and contrast opinions and reactions from those inside the critical incident boundary with those functioning as observers? It is helpful to actually plot this out with paper and pencil after the group.

Cohesion.   Rate the critical incident on the degree of group cohesion within it. Has the incident increased or decreased the sense of group involvement? The support of the group is an important sustaining factor in dealing with critical incidents.

Therapeutic factors.   Apply the therapeutic factor clusters to the event. What factors can be reinforced or invoked to assist the group process?

Precipitating event.   Look backward through the incident and try to identify when it began and what was going on at the time. The use of videotapes is helpful in catching such phenomena. The initiating circumstances not only set the tone for the incident, but may also reveal why it is important. Critical incidents often begin with a personal story by one of the members that is thematically echoed by others. Sometimes an incident will begin with an interchange between two members that has a strong, perhaps overdetermined, emotional surge behind it.

Affective tone.   Consider the principal emotional quality to the incident. Try applying the major affect states: happiness, anger, sadness, fear, disgust, surprise, and interest (52). Is there a mixture of emotional dimensions? Do these represent contradictory or incompatible dimensions? Are they expressed openly or inhibited? What is the intensity level? Emotional arousal enhances learning.

Interpersonal focus.   Identify the central interpersonal theme underlying the critical incident. Use the emotional tone and the content to place the critical incident in the Structural Analysis of Social Behavior (SASB) interactional space. This may lead to helpful speculations about its relationship to stage or role phenomena.

Developmental stage.   Compare the interactional climate and thematic focus with the stage descriptions. Do they match at an appropriate level? Has the group moved into a regressed position? Or is it testing new behavior?

Social role.   Fit role ideas onto the behaviors of the major participants in the segment. Are these their customary roles in the group, or are they trying out new ones? Role behavior may be strongly reinforced by the group and can come to shape the individual's inner sense of self. This may bring a sense of order, but can also have a restricting effect.

Interpersonal Dimensions

Once familiar with a system for applying each of these perspectives, the therapist can quickly work through a critical incident as it evolves. As a training experience, going over videotapes is invaluable in learning the process of identifying and understanding critical incidents. By focusing on these brief interpersonal vignettes, the therapist is coming close to the source of the direct impact that group events have on interpersonal learning.

By striving to understand the interpersonal dimension that lies behind or within a particular critical incident, the therapist is forced to examine group events over a brief time frame. It is easy to become fascinated by content and avoid the process. By asking the question, What are these people doing to or with each other? the actual enactment in the group of historically derived interpersonal meanings can be examined. The idea of a "corrective emotional experience" has a long history in the individual therapy literature. Analysis of critical incidents provides a parallel opportunity in the group.

One result of applying this approach to understanding a critical incident is the necessity of using the language of interactional process. Think of the difference between saying to yourself in a group, "Len is using denial," as compared to, "Len is refusing to acknowledge what Fern just said to him." The first statement would lead one toward an introspective search for the internal processes responsible for the block. The second statement might lead one to say, "Tell him again Fern, it didn't seem to penetrate, try looking him in the eye when you say it." This "massages" the interpersonal boundary between the two members and increases the affective tension that contributes to a corrective emotional experience.

A member will frequently raise an issue of concern using the language of there-and-then outside-group experiences. By translating the external story into interpersonal language, the therapist is in a better position to detect similar qualities in the group interaction. This here-and-now within-group focus intensifies the experience, makes it more real, and facilitates the working-through process of desensitization and understanding. Then the original external context can be reviewed in the light of the group experience. This may result in a "rewriting" of personal history in terms of how early events are understood. It may result in new ways of approaching current situations or the development of a different view of self.

A critical incident can usefully be considered as reflecting a state of tension between two opposing poles. This helps to "stretch out" the issue and identify the source of the creative energy underlying the incident. The idea of a psychotherapeutic dialectical process is quite valuable. Not only does it highlight the theme but it clarifies where each participant lies along the axis of tension. It is a helpful exercise to "line up" the group members between the two poles. Those in the middle of the line have less investment in the theme than those at either end. One useful therapeutic technique is to mildly caricature each pole in order to force a process of resolution to the tension: "From what you say, it sounds as if it would be impossible for you to hear yourself having such a thought." This brings us to a consideration of the idea of conflictual themes.

The Two Triangles

The Triangle of Conflict

There has been an enduring theme in the psychotherapy literature concerning the idea of thematic tension. Most approaches have

Introduction to Time-Limited Group Psychotherapy

incorporated the idea of an underlying wish, a reaction to that wish, and some attempt at a solution. Ezriel (in Scheidlinger 1980) used the terms *required relationship* that prevents the emergence of the unconscious *avoided relationship* because of fear that the latter would lead to a *calamitous relationship*. French (1954) used similar terms, the *disturbing motive* leading to a *reactive motive* that produces tension requiring a *solution*.

Malan (1979) developed the idea of a triangle of insight consisting of a defense required to control the anxiety associated with a hidden feeling or impulse. Luborsky reflects a similar idea in the CCRT model: I wish BUT . . . . The *but* describes the fears or blocks to wish fulfillment. Horowitz (1987) expanded this approach to purposefully look for several typical relationship patterns. These may reveal various options, some dysfunctional and some successful, that the patient has available in the interpersonal repertoire. Benjamin's (1974) SASB system can be used to generate a conflict score reflecting incompatible patterns within the individual or in the two-way exchanges of a relationship. SASB is commonly applied to relationships with several significant others, allowing a comparative approach similar to Horowitz's.

All of these descriptions constitute ways of describing a state of tension or conflict regarding personal issues. They all force a translation of intrapsychic phenomena into the language of relationships. This focus can be predicted to form a recurrent theme in the behavior of an individual and should recur in the here-and-now relationships of the group (53).

The triangle of conflict can be reduced to a generic format applicable to a broad set of clinical circumstances. The problematic issue (P; Figure 10-1) may be considered as either hidden or accessible to self or to others, as in the language of the Johari Window. The problematic issue is believed to result in negative or aversive consequences that produce a nonspecific reaction of anxiety (A). These consequences may also be overtly recognized or hidden from the patient's awareness. The attempted solution (S) is the resultant behavior, often the only part of the triangle that is initially visible. This solution may be considered to be adaptive or dysfunctional. The attempted solution may also be called the defense against the underlying problematic issue. The phrase *attempted solution* seems to more accurately portray the situation and encourages the clinician to align with the patient's efforts to resolve a difficult matter (54).

Behavioral and cognitive formulations can easily be placed in the structure diagrammed in Figure 10-1 as well as the psychodynamic hypotheses for which it was originally designed.

The Triangle of Person

The triangle of conflict is then placed within the *triangle of person*. In its simplest form, the triangle of person refers to relationships in current life (C; Figure 10-2), the therapeutic relationship itself (T), and past relationships, usually referring to family of origin up to adolescent years (P). The right-hand side of the triangle can be used to list important relationships from the patient's adult years.

The therapist must search each corner of the triangle of person for evidence of the impact of issues related to the theme identified in the triangle of conflict (Figure 10-3). A classic interpretation would link the emergence of the theme in current relationships to its initial development within the family of origin and then to the same pattern within the therapeutic relationship.

It is important that these connections be worked out using specific persons and specific incidents. The intent is to re-create in this space relationship memories, not generalized attitudes that may mask the reality of actual people.

Another way of looking at the triangle of person is that in real historical time the progress of events goes from the lower corner within the family of origin through a succession of relationships to the upper-right corner involving current relationships. These events may

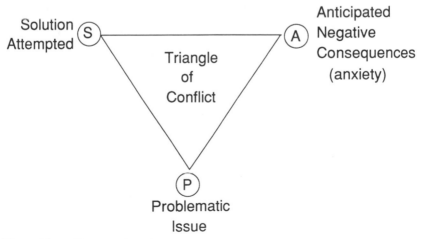

Figure 10-1.   Triangle of conflict.

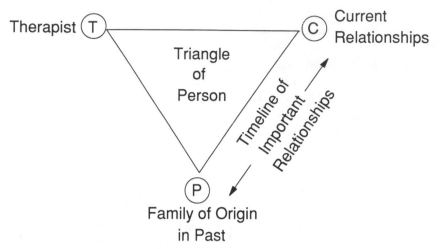

Figure 10-2.   Triangle of person.

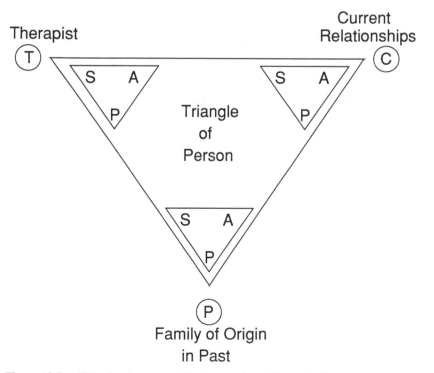

Figure 10-3.   Triangle of person with triangle of conflict applied at each corner.

be portrayed as involving a series of significant others ranged along the time line of the right side of the triangle. Any of these intervening relationships may produce ongoing effects, although it is generally assumed that earlier relationships set the basic template for understanding and reacting to interpersonal issues. Historical time then moves from current relationships to experiences within the therapy experience itself.

In therapeutic time, the sequence is often reversed. Identification of issues in current outside relationships leads to an appreciation of similar issues within the therapeutic relationship and then to connections with the past. By anchoring the learning in present relationships, both inside and outside of the therapeutic room, it is given affective power that can be used to understand the past. This makes the process of historical reconstruction a real experience, not simply a cognitive exercise. It is not clear to what extent the application to the past is necessary. People probably differ in this regard. For some, dealing with the past seems a necessary part of coming to terms with the present. For others, changing things now is all they want or need. From a therapeutic viewpoint, the goal is that future relationships are of a functional nature with a tempering of the dysfunctional patterns identified within the triangle of conflict.

In therapy groups, at the upper-left corner of the triangle of person the figure of the therapist is joined by all group members. This provides an opportunity to see any given patient at work in a number of relationships. These relationships with group members may incorporate several different interactional patterns. This recalls the idea of developing role flexibility. Rather than being locked into old fixed patterns that may have been necessary at one time, the patient can examine a series of new relationships. To link this material with stage development and social role ideas, in Figure 10-4 the other group members are figuratively identified by role labels, which have been located in the figure within the group circle in the same spatial arrangement as found in the diagram of the SASB space in Figure 5-2.

It was suggested in Chapter 6 that thought be given to trying to identify more than one interactional style for an individual. This means that the triangle of conflict might contain several relationship patterns based on previous significant others. The triangle of person can be used to try out these historic themes with those actually emerging with group members. A line can be drawn between a particular figure from the patient's history, both current and past, and a group member

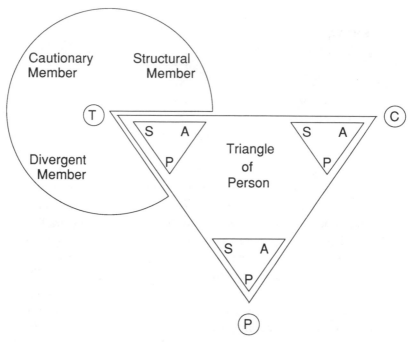

Figure 10-4. Emergence within the group of psychological material arising from triangle of conflict.

of the present. This slightly expanded version of the two triangles is shown in Figure 10-5, using the case history summarized in Table 6-1.

The therapist may use the ideas of interpersonal learning discussed earlier as a general model for inducing change. Such changes should emerge in behaviors reflecting the thematic material defined by the triangle of conflict. Fortunately, the therapist has the help of other group members. They may provide useful ways for looking at the same set of issues in different ways. By encouraging group members to think in these terms, the therapist can expand the sources of therapeutic influence.

Applying the Two Triangles to a Critical Incident

To bring this back to a particular critical incident, one may imagine the two triangles diagram of each member with the T (therapist) corner of the triangle of person applied within the group. A critical incident will produce some degree of activation for each member. The degree will vary depending on how close the critical incident theme

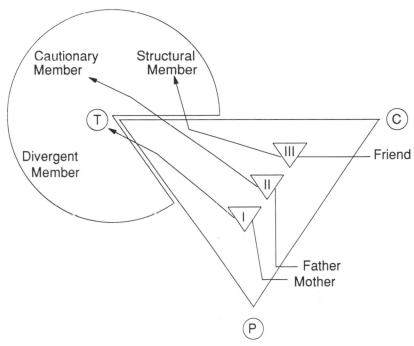

Figure 10-5. Applying the two triangles in a group context.

matches the issues in each member's triangle of conflict. This is akin
to the concept of "valency" described by Bion. The idea of ranking
the group members along the thematic dimension of the critical incident helps here. Some will be very much involved at the extremes,
others in the center might be interested but not highly reactive to the
material. In Figure 10-6, our patient is actively demonstrating a desire
for support and attention from the therapist, activating template I
from Figure 10-5 concerning an image of his childhood relationship
with his mother. This matches his CCRT wish "to be helped, protected, and comforted." The cautionary role member protests vigorously about such interpersonal neediness, perhaps in a reactive fashion to his own concerns. Note that this is the same quadrant that the
patient used to describe his father's typical reaction. The structural
and divergent members are less involved in this critical incident and
therefore are able to mediate and expand the discussion.

     It is important that the therapist have some appreciation of how
group events are impinging on each member. This system of defining
a core conflictual issue for each member facilitates a systematic
method for making these assessments. The same format can be

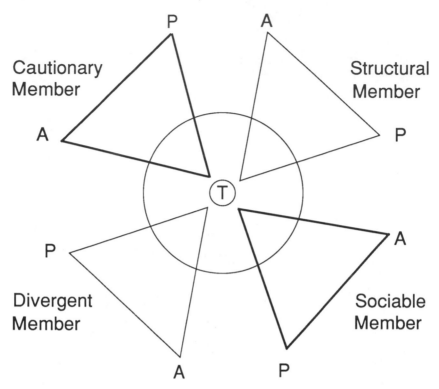

Figure 10-6. Schematic of the group during a critical incident in which the young man described in Table 6-1 activated his personal triangle of conflict issues in the lower-right quadrant. The patient across the group circle reacted strongly to this material while the others were able to function as neutral commentators.

incorporated into group records, which then form a history of the evolution and management of the triangle of conflict issues for each member as they emerge within the group context. This discussion of the theme of a critical incident can be seen as a method for applying the idea of group focal conflict. Rather than assuming that all group members are active on a particular theme at any one point in time, this approach specifically addresses the question of which members are active and which members are not. A theoretical boundary can be drawn between these two subsets of members. A fishbowl effect is created in which some members are in a position to observe and comment on the action of others. In this way, all members can be active participants in a given critical incident even though it may not be directly pertinent to them. This is a useful learning perspective for members because it encourages them to think objectively about behavior at times when they are not caught up in the action. They can eventually learn to do the same thing in regard to their own behavior.

If the interpersonal focus has been reasonably accurately defined, it should have immediate relevance to current outside relationships. By applying group learning concerned with the same focus to these real relationships, the individual can begin creating a new interpersonal climate outside the group. This exemplifies the idea of a living system contributing to the creation of its own environment. It also makes the group work directly relevant in the eyes of the members.

This material can also be viewed in terms of group developmental ideas. The work of stage 1 is primarily concerned with the current (C) corner of the triangle of person. Stage 2 tends to involve the therapist (T). Stage 3 deals with introspective issues that draw in material from the past (P). If a standard language of interpersonal dimensions is used, such as that provided by SASB, then the conflict themes within the triangle of person can be directly related to the ideas about stages and roles. This leads to the generation of hypotheses to be tested in the group concerning these underlying dimensions that link the corners of the individual's life with the circle of the group.

Summary

This chapter has moved into a psychodynamic frame of reference to deal with specific issues of interpersonal learning and insight. This process is described in terms of the mechanisms of self-disclosure, feedback, and introspection that characterize the advanced working group. The idea of critical incidents that punctuate a session is used as a focus for looking at the group therapeutic process. The focus for individual work is described in terms of an interpersonal theme organized in terms of the triangle of conflict. The triangle of conflict is applied within the temporal structure of the triangle of person. This schematic approach provides a structure for organizing the conceptualization of psychodynamic work.

CHAPTER **11**

Termination

The termination stage may occur at any point in the group's life, often because of service decisions. Inpatient groups deal with termination issues daily. Closed time-limited groups only face it once. Groups operating on a slow-open turnover system will repeatedly encounter termination issues concerning one or more members. Whenever termination does occur, it entails the same set of tasks. These will be more powerful if the group has met together for a long time. But even in quite brief group formats, termination still demands careful attention from the therapist. Just as engagement issues are of central importance to the beginning group, so ending tasks must be addressed at termination. This aspect of group work is frequently neglected.

Basic Tasks

The task at the end is threefold. The group must be incorporated as a positive and constructive experience. Each member must address issues raised by the theme of loss. Finally, material learned in the group must be applied to outside personal circumstances.

Boundary Focus

As in stage 1, the focus shifts to the external group boundary, and polarization of issues across this boundary highlights the task. During engagement, this entailed an emphasis on universality within the group that could be contrasted with outside experiences. At termination, the internal side of the boundary is emphasized by recalling group memories. This contributes to the internalization of the experience. At the same time, efforts are made to apply the therapy experience to outside situations. This assists generalization of learning.

Managing the End

There is a strong tendency in most of us to avoid the question of termination. Therapists experience this as well as group members. It is not at all uncommon for the last session to come almost as a surprise to a group, even though everyone had factual knowledge about it. The task of working through separation focuses on universal human issues that must be addressed for the therapeutic experience to be encompassed. Mann has written eloquently regarding the question of time as it applies to individual therapy. His 12-session brief psychotherapy approach is predicated on the assumption that termination work constitutes the bedrock of effective psychotherapy. This involves confronting the fact of the essential aloneness of the individual and the need to accept responsibility for self: "The major plague of human beings is a simultaneous wish to merge with another and the absolute necessity of learning to tolerate separation and loss without undue damage to feelings about oneself" (55). Rigid adherence to time boundaries forces the patient to give up unrealistic and childlike beliefs that life is eternal and that, given enough opportunity, somebody will solve all problems.

Termination puts into focus the issue of individual responsibility. By addressing and mastering such issues, the patient is able to enhance a sense of self-efficacy. The human condition entails loss and disappointment. The capacity to endure such situations constitutes a fundamental quality of satisfactory adult coping. All of these themes are present in termination discussions. They form a basis for important psychological work that must not be avoided.

The wish to deny termination is commonly expressed in talk of reunions, of continuing the group without the therapist, or of becoming a group of friends. These events seldom take place and, if they do, are usually found to be hollow and lacking in the expected reinforcement of group camaraderie. The therapist is well advised to benignly but persistently lean against these plans by focusing on their fantasy wish for ongoing nurturance and support. Although acknowledging the understandable nature of it, the unrealistic nature should also be clarified. Of course, it is not possible to prohibit such activities, but by discussing them seriously, the therapist can at least make sure that termination issues are not avoided.

The impact of termination will be in direct relationship to the degree of group cohesion. Groups that have met for only a few sessions without much personal investment will handle termination issues quickly. Longer-term groups in which learning has been emphasized will gain much from the final working-through process. There are a number of things the therapist can do to facilitate termination.

Set the date. The process of termination must be started well in advance. Themes of impending termination need to be specifically introduced if they have not already been brought up, certainly several sessions before the final date. Not all of the work of the group will be devoted to termination issues during these sessions, but it should be of increasing importance as the final session approaches. A specific termination date should be established. It is best to state this date in terms of an actual day, not in terms of how many sessions. That way there will be no doubt about its relationship to other events. The group must not simply dwindle toward its termination. With advance preparation, it may be possible to select a date on which all members will be present even if this is slightly sooner than would otherwise be the case. Groups often end in the spring or early summer when year-end events or vacations start to pose attendance problems. It is useful to review the calendar specifically with members so that to the fullest extent possible complete attendance can be expected right up to the final session. In many short-term groups, the final date is established at the outset, and such a review begins during the assessment phase. Even if this has been done, it needs to be discussed again well in advance of termination. The termination process should be addressed with the same clarity and attention to detail that was emphasized in planning for the first session.

Review of group memories. On the inside of the group boundary, a systematic review of critical incidents in the group's life and their meaning for the members helps to internalize the group experience. The therapist can assist with encouragement to think of the best memories, the worst, the most meaningful, and so on. Usually this process has a bittersweet quality to it. Early group memories rekindle the sense of expectation, almost wonder, of starting into therapy. Memories also force recognition of changes that have occurred over time.

It is particularly useful to maintain a focus on the personal learning associated with group events. The goal is not just to consolidate group memories, but also to underline coping strategies involved in them. A comparison of old and new approaches helps to highlight the changes. These reviews should not be simply a fast recall of a particular situation. The therapist can help the termination process by slowing down the memories and forcing a detailed review of their importance and the thematic material contained in them.

Grief and loss.   If the group has to any extent been a meaningful experience, its termination will reactivate general patterns of reaction to loss. Components of sadness and grief are usually contained in these associations. There will also be themes of anger or abandonment. Working through these in terms of the group itself and its individual members constitutes necessary termination work. This is not a task for the final session. It is typical of grief work that it extends over time and comes in waves. Members will experience these at home as well as in the session. Intrusive thoughts about the group are common and may appear in dreams.

Reactions to the loss of specific relationships within the group should be targeted. Some groups use formal go-arounds for this purpose in which each member addresses every other one about their experience together in the group. The purpose of this is not a maudlin display of affect, but to encourage the resolution of issues still in the air. It also helps to identify defensive use of denial. In the final session, it is useful to review how members will experience the time when the group would normally have next met. Patients may experience components of other past grief situations. Such associations are important to pursue and may be specifically sought by the therapist. The affect contained in them can be a powerful motivator for psychological mastery. The focus may begin with affect, but should also move on to a consideration of coping mechanisms in the face of loss. It is helpful to deal with these in terms of actual individuals from the patient's life, not allowing the intensity to be masked under general comments about people leaving. The task is facilitated by the review of specific memories and specific images of each person.

Transfer of learning.   Specific efforts need to be made to apply group learning to outside relationships and circumstances. As in stage 1, this "massages" the external boundary of the group. This might include a review of coping mechanisms that can be used without the physical presence of the group. Many patients find that it is useful to visualize themselves in the group setting and in their imagination to conduct a therapy session around the issue to be addressed. It is to be expected that, during therapy, psychological changes will be taking place both in terms of how individuals see themselves and how they view their relationships with others. Hopefully, these changes will have been enacted in the quality of the relationships within the group and also tried out on important relationships outside of the group. Indeed, the therapist should continuously reinforce the importance of outside application of learning throughout the group's life. During termination, the question of generalization of learning comes specifically into focus.

One particular aspect of this transfer of learning involves a prediction into the future. The members can be asked to think of stressful situations and how they will be addressed. They can work through such events and try to predict the nature of the difficulties they will experience and the sort of reactions they are likely to have. Adaptive coping strategies can be rehearsed. This continues the work of incorporation by reinforcing behaviors that will help to maintain change in the future.

Final ceremonies.   Many groups will include some ritualistic element to the final session. At a minimum, this might include a go-around of good-byes by each member to each of the others, including the therapist. These are not intended to be perfunctory statements. Each member should be encouraged to address specific memories about each of the others, events in their relationship in the group, and thoughts about change, future goals, and so on.

Termination rituals may include standing and forming a ring of joined hands for a moment of contemplation. Some groups mimic the funeral ritual of sharing food. Symbolic termination activities are perfectly acceptable and indeed can be quite powerful. The process of planning for such events is as important as what actually takes place. The therapist needs to be sure that such activities come after the termination process has been worked through and signify its end, not an avoidance of the task.

Social Roles

Members will address the termination task in their customary fashion. The stress of termination will often be revealed in a degree of regression into stereotypic character behavior. This might be noted by the therapist so that it is not interpreted by the members as a sign of lack of progress. It is typically a short-lived phenomenon. Similarly, a recurrence of symptoms is common. Interpretive linkage of these to termination reactions is helpful. It may foster a constructive attitude in which symptoms are seen as resulting from specific situations, not as independent and mysterious phenomena.

The sociable role members will find termination the most difficult. They are likely to be the ones most interested in alumni get-togethers. They can be encouraged to use the good-bye statements to think through the issues, not just react. The divergent role members will also regret leaving, though they may not admit it openly. Special care that they are acknowledged is useful. The structural role members can be counted on to lead the discussion about outside application and personal goals. The cautionary role members are in a position to help the group clarify the importance of individual responsibility for one's life. For these last two roles, termination carries less of a threat, but the therapist should be sure that their reactions are probed beneath the surface acceptance.

Predictable Problems

Denial of termination. The careful review of the termination date mentioned above is not just an exercise in therapeutic compulsivity. By establishing a specific date, it is possible to focus on termination work. This is a task that is frequently avoided. It is not uncommon to encounter therapists reacting with surprise to find that there are only two sessions left and termination has not yet been discussed. Quite simply, this is inadequate.

Therapists have a clear responsibility for polarizing termination issues and must be held accountable if this process does not occur. Group members as well as therapists are often reluctant to address these matters. Pressing group issues often seem to emerge that demand attention but actually serve to avoid dealing with termination matters. As part of this termination focus, the therapist should repeatedly reinforce the expectation that all members will attend all final sessions.

Premature termination.   Members having difficulty with separation issues may begin to miss sessions or actually terminate early. This allows them to retain some sense of control over termination and in the process avoid dealing with its implications. This may apply particularly to members who have had trouble accommodating to losses in the past, such as the early loss of a parent. Patients who have developed considerable dependency on the group may also try to handle this through premature terminations. The therapist should be alert to such issues and try to forestall them by raising the question of such possibilities for discussion.

Termination of an individual member.   This book has dealt primarily with time-limited groups that begin and end as a unit. The termination arrangements are built into the package and are thus in one sense easier to address. Inevitably, individual members may for one reason or another be unable to continue. The above guidelines must be addressed in regard to that one member. This not only manages the termination process for that member but also serves as a clear marker of the external boundary. The group must restructure itself without that member. Indeed, a useful theme is to review the role that member has played in the group, what it has meant to the individual, and what it will mean to the group not to have that person performing those role functions.

   Not uncommonly, a member indicates the intention to leave the group to the therapist in a private manner or at the end of the session. Should the member be expected to return for a final session and "say good-bye"? If the member is terminating after only a few sessions, as discussed in Chapter 8, such an event is usually neither helpful to the group nor therapeutic for the individual. If the person leaving has been a well-established member of the group, the termination process must not be avoided. The member should be strongly advised to return for at least one final session. This is particularly important if the member's decision to leave has been precipitated by a specific critical incident, as discussed in the next section.

   The termination of a member forces the group to reorganize as a system. This inevitably causes at least temporary regression and a drop in group morale. The therapist must be prepared to adjust to the emergence of early group phenomena characteristic of the engagement and differentiation stages. This is usually brief, but may become serious if the group has been having chronic problems with dropouts or poor attendance.

Negative terminations.   Most situations of negative termination involve group-level issues. Often these are of a scapegoating nature.
Therefore, letting them pass without close examination may be setting the stage for a future repetition with another targeted member. In
a final session, it may be possible to reframe the circumstances so that
the departing member will have a positive rationale for the process.

The group members also have something to learn by a review of
such situations. If the precipitating critical incident involved an attack,
criticism, or rejection, members may be harboring guilt about it. An
opportunity to explore this may reveal personal issues that contributed to the attack in the first place. The goal of having a member
return to terminate is not necessarily to pressure him or her into
continuing. Important work can be accomplished for all parties
whether or not the decision is reconsidered.

Members leaving a group in a negative frame of mind are at risk
of undoing therapeutic work. When people look back on the group
experience, they view it through the terminating experience. If this is
unpleasant or unresolved, they may be unable to internalize what
might have been therapeutic and constructive. Efforts to work
through termination issues may therefore be quite therapeutic both to
the individual and to the group. The question of negative effects is
discussed at more length in Chapter 13.

Satisfaction with therapy.   Some patients, though symptomatically
improved, may feel dissatisfied with the group experience. They may
handle the stress of termination with the idea that they never had the
individual attention they had sought. The benefits of group versus
individual therapy was one topic in the pretherapy preparation material. The same issues come into focus at the time of termination.
Attitudes about having had group therapy, and perhaps time-limited
group therapy to boot, should be openly explored. Into this discussion,
the therapist can usefully introduce the idea that in fact the members
have improved, that no therapy is going to handle all personal issues,
and that they have acquired tools to use in their ongoing adjustment.
The therapist can reinforce the idea that patients continue to improve
in the year or two after therapy as they apply what they have learned.
This information is helpful in allowing patients to get a sense of
perspective on their situation. It need not be presented apologetically,
but rather as a clear statement of therapeutic confidence (56).

Personal reactions of the therapist.   The therapist may experience
reluctance to deal with termination matters openly. There may be

many reasons for this. Beginning therapists may wonder if they have "done enough" for the patients and feel that any thought of ending the group is tantamount to abandonment. Some therapists become overly involved in assisting patients and find it difficult to relinquish control and allow autonomy. Such issues are brought clearly into focus at the point of termination. Therapists who are overly supportive may fear the negative interpretation they assume patients will give to the idea of stopping. For some therapists, group termination may activate personal experiences of loss.

Therapists need to pay careful attention to the manner in which they approach the time of termination. They may without fully realizing find themselves colluding with patient resistance. The structure provided by the tasks outlined above will help to alleviate such tendencies.

Summary

The work of termination helps to round off the group experience so that it can be incorporated. The underlying principle to the various strategies outlined in this chapter is that termination must be openly discussed as an important part of the therapeutic process. It is easy for this work to be postponed or avoided. The therapist must be alert to personal reactions that align with patient resistance to this task.

CHAPTER **12**

Therapist Style

This chapter addresses the activities of the therapist. To this point, most attention has been paid to understanding the phenomena of groups with only anecdotal mention of what to do. A number of dimensions of the therapist's general style are discussed, including some simple techniques that form a base for the use of more complex therapeutic interventions. The most accurate and sophisticated interpretation will fail if the group environment has not been carefully prepared. This chapter constitutes a summary of therapeutic activities that is applicable to all groups. The next chapter goes into more detail about the approach to making psychodynamic interventions.

Basic Therapeutic Dimensions

Numerous studies of group therapist behavior have identified a few basic characteristics that correlate with successful outcome. These dimensions provide useful guidelines for a new group therapist who is developing a personal style. Of course, the impact of leader behavior on patient outcome is modified by member-to-member experiences. But the therapist is in a position to exert considerable influence on the sort of group climate that emerges (57).

Caring and Support

One of the most critical therapist attributes is a basic attitude of positive regard and concern toward patients. This theme goes far back in the psychotherapy research literature as a necessary condition for effective therapy. It is connected to Frank's (1973) emphasis on the importance of hope and the power of a positive relationship to enhance a sense of self-efficacy. This basic "therapeutic attitude" does not imply giving in to all patient demands, nor approving of all patient behavior. It does embody a central ethic of the helping professions that their function is to support mastery, not judge deficiencies.

Carl Rogers considered several components to be essential for effective therapy:

1. *Nonpossessive warmth* refers to a caring attitude that is not controlling. It is somewhat paradoxical that the caricature of the Rogerian therapist is one who exudes a "taking care of" attitude.
2. *Accurate empathy* concerns the therapist's attempts to understand how patients see their personal and interpersonal world, so that the therapist is able to predict how they are likely to view events. This does not imply agreement, nor even a feeling of kinship. Such responses would be better termed *sympathy*.
3. *Genuineness* describes the therapist acting as a real person responding in a personal fashion with some degree of spontaneity. It does not preclude the therapist using clinical judgment to filter the strength of responses.
4. *Unconditional positive regard* refers to an attitude that patients are attempting to cope as well as they can and that their efforts therefore should be seen as constructive even if misguided. The therapist is seen as aligning with the patient against the psychopathology.

Rogers considered these qualities to be both necessary and sufficient for effective therapy. Contemporary research suggests that they are very important in establishing a working environment, but that additional factors of technique need also to be considered. The term *therapeutic alliance* is now used to describe many of the same features (58).

Cognitive Understanding

The second broad area of therapist responsibility is to promote an understanding of the problematic behavior. This refers to a general quality of understanding the rationale for difficulties and for the methods proposed to deal with them. It is important in all types of therapy.

Some studies suggest that the content of the proposed rationale is less important than the fact that there is one. A framework for understanding permits a sense of cognitive mastery over the situation. This focus on the cognitive dimension of therapy is an important and pervasive therapist activity that has been found to correlate with positive outcome. Much of the material in Chapter 10 on the working group deals with ways of establishing a focus for addressing the cognitive understanding of presenting issues (59).

Therapist Control

Group therapists are often concerned about the question of responsibility for initiating group activity. Patients will come with the plausible statement, "Since you are the leader, lead us." This is a role expectation trap that requires adroit management. A leadership profile that is too low will leave a group feeling lost and demoralized, a high level of control will inhibit responses.

The optimal degree of leader control is related to the goals of the group and to the capabilities of the members. Therapists tend to underestimate the capabilities of group members. They slip into a style of leadership that involves a greater degree of management than necessary. This is not to deny the ultimate professional responsibility that always lies behind therapeutic decisions, but rather the question of how much to control the group process.

Control may be exerted in many fashions. The most obvious way is by structuring group activities. For example, a specific task may be prescribed such as a go-around of responses or role-playing or psychodrama activities. Less obvious control may be exerted by the therapist through a subtle molding of process events. For example, some therapists establish a style in which most patient statements are directed to them and are answered by them. Thus, group communication channels are restricted. Control may also be exerted by the use of interpretive statements that serve to bring closure to an issue. Through the use of summarizing or absolute conclusions, the therapist may "put the lid on" further discussion.

All of these interventions may be quite correct in terms of the content expressed. However, the interpersonal process message is that the leader is in charge (and the members are not). An overly active and controlling therapist produces passive and submissive group members. Such members are not only more likely to have lower levels of initiation in the group but also will approach their own personal problem resolution with a greater degree of passivity, expecting answers from the therapist.

The effects of control follow a curvilinear model. Some degree of control stabilizes a group and provides a structure around which it can function effectively. As the level of control increases, a point is reached where it becomes an inhibiting and stultifying influence. Control is most constructive when it is directed at creating conditions for the enactment of therapeutic factors, including the maintenance of a task focus. By developing a therapeutic milieu, the therapist is indirectly influencing the members through its impact. The individual member is free to use this environment for the exploration of personally important themes. This shaping task may be accomplished by quite subtle techniques of reinforcement, modeling, and quiet suggestions. Once important content themes are established, the therapist may be of assistance in reinforcing a focus on them. The therapist is in a position to say, in effect, "This is the material you wanted to work on, I will try to make sure it does not get avoided."

The group developmental perspective suggests that a certain amount of therapist initiation is appropriate in the early stages of group. During the engagement stage, the therapist has a responsibility to the group to promote the development of an effective and cohesive system. This responsibility should be tapered so that the members may feel confident of initiating leadership challenge during the differentiation stage. The eventual goal is the development of a working group that will assume much of the leadership function for promoting therapeutic change. This theme of the therapist using the group as the agent of change runs through much of this book.

More structure is appropriate when the interactional capacity of the group members is limited. Groups for patients exhibiting the negative symptoms of schizophrenia do better with an active and structuring therapist. Inpatient groups with acutely ill patients require structure to maintain a pragmatic work focus. Nonetheless, the therapist must be aware that the more control provided, the less autonomy is possible for the group members. As a general principle, control by the therapist should be kept to the lowest level that is compatible with maintaining a functional group (60).

Stimulation of Emotional Arousal

Some therapeutic activities act as a stimulant to high emotional arousal in the group. Such therapists are personally very involved in the group process. They use high levels of therapist self-disclosure, high levels of therapist control, and a tendency to be aggressively intrusive into patients' emotional lives. They exhort the members to open up like the leader is doing. This constellation of features describes charismatic leaders who by the force of their personality and demanding techniques will pull people into their influence. As we will see in a section in Chapter 13 on negative effects, such techniques may have beneficial results for some patients but carry a greater risk of negative effects. Some members in such groups report that they regretted saying too much, or that they were attacked by the leader or by others acting under the leader's suggestion (61).

Effect on Outcome

The above four aspects of leader style—caring and support, cognitive understanding, therapist control, and stimulation of emotional arousal—account for a considerable effect on outcome. Figure 12-1 shows these connections. Caring and cognitive work have a direct effect on outcome—the more of these qualities the better. Control and emotional stimulation have a curvilinear relationship.

Outcome Success

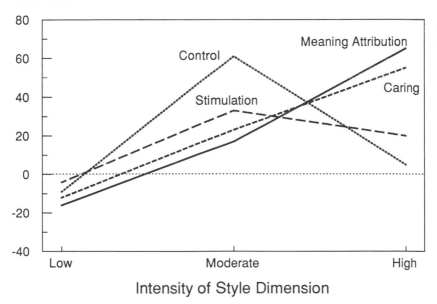

Figure 12-1. Relationship between outcome and four therapist style dimensions.

Groups with low levels of leader control become disorganized and lose their task focus. High levels of control have an inhibiting effect on group participation. Groups with low levels of leader stimulation tend to be flat and uninteresting to the members. High stimulation levels produced active and exciting groups, but also a higher number of casualties.

Therapist Activity Level

One way of characterizing therapist behavior is simply to count the number of interventions made in a given time period. This is not the same thing as control, although they may be related. A relatively silent therapist may, by an austere attitude, be quite controlling. An active and nervous therapist may not be taken seriously. There may be vast differences in regard to activity levels. Some therapists are likely to speak no more than half a dozen times during a session. Others participate at a rate of several times per minute. The level of therapist activity will vary for numerous reasons:

1. *Group goals.*   Therapists are more active in groups designed for specific behaviorally oriented goals. Such groups generally do not use interpersonal learning as the central therapeutic process. These types of groups include social skills groups, psychoeducational programs, and groups being conducted according to cognitive-behavioral strategies.
2. *Group development.*   The functions of the designated leader must shift as the group matures. In the early stages, greater leader activity and a modest amount of direction is quite appropriate. As the group moves into working stages, there should be higher expectations for the initiation of group momentum to arise from the members. An underactive leader may frustrate the group excessively in the first few sessions, whereas an overactive therapist may inhibit group development at a later point.
3. *Critical incidents.*   The level of therapist activity may need to increase sharply if a potentially damaging situation develops. Therapists may be reluctant to change their style because of general principles about letting the group assume responsibility for the therapeutic momentum. Such good intentions do not relieve the therapist of responsibility. It is appropriate for the therapist to say openly that he or she is taking over control of the group for a while to help resolve an impasse. This transmits a message to the mem-

bers that they can try out risky behaviors knowing that there is a safety net.

4. *Therapist anxiety.*   Some therapists increase their activity when anxious; others decrease it. In either direction, such responses can have an adverse effect on the group. The overactive therapist may need to devise control strategies, such as inserting delays before making any comment. The underactive therapist can practice interventions of a minor nature at regular intervals to get practice. It is the responsibility of the therapist to monitor his or her activity level and assess the effect it is having on the group.

The level of activity transmits implicit messages regarding the locus of help. Even statements that appear to be noncontrolling imply that the therapist's efforts are required. To use group mechanisms most effectively, the therapist should defer to group initiatives unless there are clear reasons for not doing so. Before each intervention the therapist might ask, "Is this really necessary?" "Can the group get to this point by itself?" If there is any doubt in the answers, then a short delay might resolve the question. Similarly, interventions should generally be kept brief. Often a well-chosen sentence is adequate. If the contribution exceeds a brief paragraph, it is probably becoming redundant.

Operant Conditioning and Modeling

In Chapters 2 and 3, the use of operant conditioning techniques and modeling of desired behaviors was discussed. These influencing processes will be going on whether or not the therapist is specifically aware of them and will play a significant role in molding the group atmosphere. It is useful to try to bring them into full awareness. Members are acutely attuned to the nuances of therapist behavior. Glances toward or away, nods, aha's, and approving chuckles will all serve as effective reinforcers. A kicking foot, a clenched fist, or a fleeting look of concern will all register. An impassive therapist face that reveals no reaction to group events models an inhibited affective style. The beginning therapist should pay close attention to these behavioral issues. They can then be brought under conscious control and used systematically for their effects. This is not to deny spontaneity or to promote a highly manipulative approach, but the therapist must be prepared to apply clinical judgment in filtering responses in the service of therapeutic goals.

Use of Homework

One general task for the therapist is to systematically promote application of therapeutic work. Outcome is improved when group learning is actively applied to outside circumstances. Evidence that patients have been thinking about issues raised in therapy during the intervening time between sessions is a good prognostic sign. The importance of continuing group work throughout the week should be stressed beginning in pretherapy preparation and regularly throughout therapy. Sometimes this psychological homework is extended into dreams that are directly related to therapy issues or the group itself. Such dream material is usefully explored in the group, with an opportunity for all members to associate to the themes in it. In this fashion, it is treated as any other manifestation of process reaction.

Therapeutic homework not only maintains the continuity of therapy, it carries an implicit message that the patient must shoulder a portion of the therapeutic responsibility. When patients claim that they have no recall of a preceding session, this should be taken as clear and specific evidence of resistance and addressed as such. Note should be taken of the issues involved in the "forgotten" episode, and a watch made for their reappearance in the present session. This almost always will occur, and with it a gradual return of the hidden material. This undramatic approach to the mysterious amnesia is usually more productive than exhortations to remember.

Another category of homework relates to specific behavioral tasks. Different types of therapy may use homework in varying ways. Members of groups with a strong behavioral component will feel comfortable with specific homework assignments to be reported back to the group. Counting or recording specific behaviors in diaries almost always results in a marked drop in their frequency. This, however, is only one end of a general expectation that patients will begin trying out new ways of coping from an early point in the therapeutic process. This expectation should be verbalized in early sessions, and evidence of such applications should be specifically reinforced. It is useful to recall from time to time that the purpose of therapy is not to change within the sessions, although that is usually a good sign. The purpose is to alter outside relationships and circumstances. It is a fantasy born of resistance for patients to anticipate that they will get better during therapy and then change their behavior afterward. The process of applied change must begin promptly and continue regularly.

The therapist should carefully monitor such applications outside the group. These can result in unfortunate situations if the patient attempts to apply group behaviors inappropriately. In general, psychotherapy groups deal with issues involved in close relationships, not necessarily those that pertain to the working place or an impersonal public setting. Patients may misjudge the timing of their application attempts and try out behaviors suitable for close relationships with their employer, with unfortunate results. For example, a young woman caught in a marriage to a highly domineering man resolved to become more assertive, but she tried this out first with her boss and was promptly fired.

Therapist Self-disclosure

Another important aspect of therapist style is that of self-disclosure. For practical purposes, it is most useful to look at self-disclosure in terms of two categories of information: 1) revelation of personal information or beliefs and 2) responses to group events (62).

There is reasonable agreement in the literature that patients may want to know about their therapist's personal lives, but that in fact they do not really expect this. Considerable personal self-disclosure will blur the distinction between the role of designated leader and that of group member. The role of designated leader provides a symbolic figure with whom important psychotherapeutic work can occur. To abdicate this position deprives the group of these experiences. An exception to this may be some reference to general human experiences that serves to align the therapist with patient experiences. These may include such things as adjusting to the death of a parent, a sense of accomplishment at graduation, or the pride and pleasure one might take in children. Such global statements are more testimonials to the human condition than to specific therapist experiences. Therapists who find themselves straying into personal self-disclosure should question their motivations. Such material will probably not be therapeutic and may represent an attempt to reject the responsibilities of leadership or avoid group processes such as therapist challenge. This is related to the issues raised in the next chapter concerning therapist neutrality.

The matter of therapist self-disclosure in regard to events happening within the group is more complex. The first thing to bear in mind is that any statement by the therapist that implies a personal response or evaluation of group events will have a strong impact on the members. The therapist should evaluate and screen the level of responses before committing them to words. An appropriate guideline is to always delay and dampen the level of responses, knowing that they will be magnified in importance by the members. This is not intended to violate the idea of therapist spontaneity or genuineness, only to monitor and use it therapeutically.

Such responses by the therapist may be used specifically to reinforce group norms or to mold interactional style. They may be part of a general supportive and encouraging approach. Statements of therapist approval are more appropriate in groups with more socially dysfunctional members. The therapist must be careful to attend to all group members. Any hint that the therapist is "playing favorites" can be quite destructive. This may occur in a subtle fashion if the therapist becomes influenced by group dynamics that promote or criticize the role of a particular member.

Responses that lie on the negative side of the interactional spectrum may be interpreted by patients as attack or blame and should not be part of the therapeutic repertoire. These seldom have a positive effect and serve only to further alienate or shut down group interaction. This does not mean that the therapist might not on occasion align with a group member's perception that some of his or her behaviors are unwarranted, but care should be taken that such alignment is about specific behaviors, not about the person in general. In Chapter 13, the use of confrontation is discussed. It is important that this technique be seen as a technical maneuver, not a vehicle for personal attack. This is a boundary line that may easily be breached.

Managing Group Interaction

Monitoring Group Structure

Chapter 3 contains a simple structural diagram of the group and its members (Figure 3-1). It is useful for the therapist to regularly scan the group with that diagram in mind.

1. *External group boundary.*   Is the external boundary of the group intact? Is there a sense of cohesion? Is the group interacting as a system?
2. *Therapist-member boundary.*   What is the state of the boundary between the therapist subsystem and the rest of the group? Are

there sources of tension that have not been addressed? Is the role of the leader in balance regarding levels of activity and control?

3. *Member-member boundaries.* Are there issues between any two members that have come up in the session, but have not yet been addressed?

4. *Subgrouping.* Are there particular subgroups that need to be identified?

5. *Distribution of participation.* Are there some members who have not been participating? Is the action getting sidetracked onto a small number of vocal members?

6. *Internal issues.* What is the internal state of each member of the group at this point? Are the therapist and the group too preoccupied with the person speaking to recognize other issues going on within individuals? How does the material being addressed in the group have reference to each member in terms of that person's own past experience and therapeutic issues?

Fortunately, all issues do not need to be addressed at once. Themes that are missed for the moment will return if they are important. But a fast structural scan may alert the therapist to work that is waiting to be done. In particular, it may draw attention to group issues that have become lost because of preoccupation with individual matters and vice versa.

Attending to Process

The therapist must strive to understand the interactional process going on in the group. This involves a constant struggle to avoid being caught up solely in the content of the material. The therapist might practice moving in and out of the group process. At times, the therapist will be very much an interactional member of the group, but must be able to back out of the group and view it as an observer. This should happen every few minutes during a group so that it becomes second nature to think on a double-track system. At one level, the therapist is attending to the words and the content themes while at the same time looking at the process through which the material is being presented or handled. This involves addressing the question, Why are these persons talking to each other in this fashion right now?

The therapist should resist the temptation to offer quick interpretive explanations. The initial task is to describe what is happening. For this purpose, the use of a systematic approach is very helpful. The interpersonal descriptive system provided by Structural Analysis of Social Behavior (SASB) is one that can be easily applied for clinical use. The focus is not the content of the material being discussed but the process between the members. The process often throws new light on the meaning of the content. In some ways, it is easier to do this in groups than in individual therapy, because the therapist can back out of the action inconspicuously and watch how members are dealing with each other. Reviewing videotapes of sessions is a great method to develop this perceptual skill.

Using Social Role Concepts

The usefulness of the idea of social role as a bridge between individual behavioral patterns and group needs was discussed in Chapter 5. The idea of social roles can also be incorporated into some interesting and powerful therapeutic techniques. These are based on the idea of developing role flexibility—the capacity to adopt different types of relationship styles as circumstances warrant. The therapist can promote the safe exploration of role behavior in the group under controlled circumstances as a way of desensitizing patients to antici-pated fears. The nature of the role adopted is generally directly related to the therapeutic task. The work component is not limited to trying out role behavior but to carefully considering the reactions this gener-ates. Bear in mind that there is usually a direct connection between conflictual issues and the social role adopted.

A few therapeutic strategies to consider are presented here, but the scope of this approach is limited only by the therapist's creativity. The therapist may ask patients to consider a different view of them-selves by trying out one of the following instructions:

1. *Be the opposite of your usual self.*   Try out a style drawn from the opposite side of the SASB space. If you are excessively warm and nurturing, try being rather schizoid. If you analyze everything to death, play at being impulsive. Sometimes the opposite role is too big a step, and warming up to it by moving just a little around the SASB circle should be tried first. The positive and trusting sociable role member might try making a critical and blaming statement; or the analytic and cognitive structural role member may be asked to use only emotional language.
2. *Be someone else.*   This is a subtle variant on the first. The model

to be imitated may be someone outside the group, or even better, one of the group members. This approach may have the advantage of seeming to be less threatening.

3. *Become your own caricature.* Try exaggerating yourself. This is a paradoxical intervention commonly used in family therapy.
4. *Watch yourself.* Have someone else play your role in a typical situation. The same effect may be achieved through use of video playback.

These sorts of miniexercises encourage a flexibility in conceptualizing behavior, but do so in a relatively nonthreatening manner. After the exercise, serious applications can be considered.

Summary

This chapter has identified a number of therapist style characteristics and techniques. These provide guidelines that therapists can use in considering typical group behaviors. The overall effect of therapist style is multidimensional, residing both in personal characteristics and specific techniques. The dimensions described here can be used to evaluate and modify therapeutic behavior in all types of groups. These characteristics may be used in different combinations depending on the nature of the group, but together form a reasonable language for conceptualizing the therapeutic task.

CHAPTER 13

The Therapeutic Encounter

This chapter addresses in greater detail the relationship between the therapist and the group members. The material applies to all groups but is most specifically relevant to groups using more expressive and intrusive techniques. It begins with some issues related to the personality of the therapist, followed by more complex matters regarding the therapeutic stance of neutrality. Interventions are considered in terms of two major categories: clarification and confrontation. The chapter ends with a review of the types of situations that can lead to negative effects. These are regularly reported by patients in groups, and the therapist needs to be in a position to identify risky situations.

Personality of the Therapist

Psychotherapy comes more naturally to some than others. Despite fully adequate training opportunities, some professionals find it difficult to become comfortable in a situation that involves an approach that is primarily verbal and interactional. These patterns frequently become even more evident in family or group therapy that requires the therapist to deal with a larger system. There are some therapist qualities that enhance an adaptation to a systems approach.

A willingness to show a desire to help others and demonstrate empathic listening is fundamental. Note that these qualities must be enacted to be effective. Even in the presence of the best intentions, a reticence to become overtly involved will act as an inhibiting influence on psychotherapeutic work. It is helpful to have curiosity about understanding interpersonal processes. This stands in some contrast to approaches that focus primarily on solving specific problems. Of course, problems must be solved, but having some satisfaction out of the process of doing so helps. Effective use of process learning is enhanced by a spark of creativity and comfort in risking spontaneous responses. A small touch of the theatrical is not out of place in groups.

The group therapist is in a very real sense on public display. It is important that the therapist therefore learn to monitor and govern nonverbal reactions. This does not imply a frozen style, but rather the appearance of competence and self-assurance. Therapists may find themselves overreacting to group pressures by becoming either excessively active or withdrawing into silence. A particularly difficult task is to handle group hostility with equanimity. The power of this may at times seem overwhelming, yet the management of hostility is an important task for both the group and the individual member.

Psychotherapy, and work in the field of psychiatric care in general, requires the ability to tolerate ambiguity. It often takes time to gain a full appreciation of the behavioral phenomena presented by our patients. We are dependent for most of our diagnostic information on observing behavior and listening to what patients report. Information obtained in this fashion is significantly influenced by the relationship features of the situation. This includes the interviewing or interactional skills of the professional. Sometimes time is the only way to clarify confusing or contradictory impressions. These problems are particularly pronounced in the group psychotherapy situation. The therapist has the difficult task of adhering to a double agenda. There is the technical job of making sense of what is going on in the group and devising and implementing intervention strategies. At the same time, the therapist needs to remain open to picking up subtle and poorly formulated thoughts from the members. This requires a free-floating attention that is not anchored to specific immediate goals and a willingness to wait without taking immediate action. Therapists who are too procedure oriented may become out of touch with important group or individual processes. Therapists who are sensitive and responsive may find themselves losing track of necessary therapeutic tasks. It is useful for the therapist to practice jumping back and forth between these two aspects: one primarily cognitive, the other essentially experiential. There is need for both the right and left cerebral hemispheres to be at work.

The intent of a psychotherapeutic approach is to foster patient autonomy to the fullest extent possible, and through that to promote a sense of self-efficacy. It is essential that the therapist be comfortable in allowing an appropriate relinquishment of control. In group therapy, it is impossible, and would be counterproductive if it were possible, to tightly manage the group process. Certainly the therapist is in a position to influence the group culture, but that is an indirect function. The therapist must use judgment in assessing the level of autonomy appropriate for a given patient. To encourage too much may be dangerous or lead to an experience of failure; to foster too little impedes possible progress.

Therapist Neutrality

The therapist must learn to adopt a position of neutrality in the approach to the patient. The therapeutic task is to address the psychopathology underlying dysfunctional behavior. To find oneself reacting strongly to a patient indicates a loss of perspective and will have a significant impact on the therapeutic process. This is of particular concern when the intention is to use interpretations based on the patient's relationship with the therapist. In individual therapy, it is expected that the therapeutic relationship is not a real one, even though that may be desired. In groups, there is scope for greater imprecision about this.

The intent of therapist neutrality is to preserve the "as if" quality of the therapeutic situation. Control of personal responses helps to maintain a frame around this artificial situation. Indeed, it is important that it is never a real relationship, but rather a therapeutic context in which one is helping, the other being helped. The interpersonal needs of the patient as expressed toward the therapist are not gratified, but examined. The task of the therapist is to accept the patient's material and assist in the process of understanding it. This demands that the therapist be loyal to the therapeutic system, not aligned for or against the patient.

These comments do not imply that the therapist need be unresponsive, e.g., only a blank screen or a reflecting mirror. An empathic attitude remains important as well as warmth and concern. However, an overly reactive stance renders the therapist vulnerable to being misinterpreted and may foster patient attempts to negotiate special alliances. The goal might be described as detachment without insensibility (63).

It is easy to lose neutrality in groups. The group will exert a powerful suction on the therapist to join with the members' views regarding difficulties and ideal solutions. Several issues can be identified that might lead to a loss of therapist neutrality.

Denial of separateness.   The therapist's situation is in many ways a lonely one. The therapist may try to break out of this self-imposed role. A group setting may intensify this type of reaction. Everyone else is relishing the fruits of universality, and the therapist must watch as an onlooker, forbidden to fully partake.

Avoiding specific transferences.   Therapists may find themselves reacting to particular expectations of the group. They may want to protest their lack of perfection when being idealized in stage 1. They may want to plead their essential goodness when they are the subject of group criticism in stage 2. Such reactions may represent personal areas of relative vulnerability for the therapist.

Therapist self-centeredness.   The therapist may experience some need to promote a particular view of life, or to develop a group of personal followers. This not only leads to undue control, it violates the technical task of understanding, not determining, the direction of change. Some therapists find it difficult to refrain from an excess of exhibitionistic behavior, going well beyond the "small touch of the theatrical" mentioned earlier. This may entertain a group, and indeed make converts, but it undermines the importance of the members themselves doing the hard work.

Personal reactions (countertransference).   The question of therapist reactions to psychodynamic material is too broad for an extended discussion here. The literature on individual psychotherapy has much to offer in this regard. In groups, a powerful and rather primitive set of pressures can develop, such as those described by Bion. These are rooted in basic human concerns for acceptance, recognition, protection, and self-esteem. Therapists may find themselves reacting to such material in an uncomfortably strong manner. Coming out of a group session, the therapist may realize that the nature of an intervention was uncalled for or overdetermined. Intrusive thoughts about the group between sessions may indicate that an area of personal sensitivity or vulnerability has been approached. In such situations, some form of supervisory consultation is indicated. This may be of a formal nature or simply a discussion with a knowledgeable colleague.

Because strong personal responses are common in groups, it is important that the group therapist have a sound background in individual psychotherapy and some exposure to experiential group training. At the very least, this will alert the clinician to problematic areas or issues. If these continue to interfere with sound clinical judgment, then a more formal personal training or therapeutic opportunity may be of value.

Making Skillful Interventions

Clarification Versus Confrontation

One basic way of thinking about therapist interventions is to divide them into clarification or confrontation categories. Both approaches may be used to address focal issues. Clarification seeks more information about the issue or situation. Confrontation draws attention to some aspect of the situation and offers a direct or implicit interpretation as to its meaning or significance. Both techniques introduce a component of structure and control into the process by their focusing action. However, they differ in the way they do this (64).

The basic intent of clarification is to promote an opportunity for a response that is determined by the patient. This enhances patient autonomy and also promotes an alignment with the patient's inner world that enhances empathic bonds. By seeking more information, clarification allows situations to be understood in more complex ways. In Chapter 10, the mechanisms of self-disclosure and interpersonal feedback were described. In a group situation, this process allows enormous scope for effective use of clarification questions. When properly applied, clarification leads to more effective conflict resolution: "I may not entirely agree but at least I understand your situation better." The therapist does not need to feel compelled to come up with accurate interpretations that will produce immediate insight. By massaging the interaction with clarification questions, the therapist is promoting the interpersonal learning cycle.

The goals of confrontation techniques are similar in nature. In a formal sense, confrontation challenges an opinion or a response or offers a new explanation that links various issues from the past to the present or across several circumstances. In either case, it is offered to promote a new awareness and thus "confronts" the patient's existing understanding of self or situation with an alternative possibility. Confrontation should not be seen as necessarily an adversarial process with an implied contest of wills. It may become that, but it is better to think of it in a technical fashion as a way of opening new channels for thought. This approach is different from clarification because the answer is implied in the confrontational message. There must of necessity be a comparison of two viewpoints. This makes it easier for the patient to accept or reject the suggestion.

Recent studies in individual therapy suggest that confrontation techniques in general do not promote the therapeutic task as effectively as clarification. Confrontations are followed by more defended responses indicating closure on the subject. However, confrontation techniques do result in further exploration when the patient is already in an open and accessible state. In other words, when the patient is already searching for alternative explanations, interpretations may be constructively received. This is in keeping with a long psychotherapeutic tradition that emphasizes the importance of timing when making interventions. The idea of looking for patient openness is a useful clinical guideline for judging when to use confrontations. It may save the therapist from getting caught in nonproductive efforts to hammer home a point when the patient is quite impervious to penetration (65).

Clarification and confrontation have interesting differences when placed within the Structural Analysis of Social Behavior (SASB) space. Clarification interventions are primarily located in the upper-right quadrant. They are positively motivated and ask for a patient response that enhances autonomy: "Can you explore a bit more what you meant by that idea of fearing to get close? [Feel free to open up.]" Confronting interpretations that are presented as ideas or suggestions for consideration also lie in this area: "Have you ever considered that there may be a connection between your present fears and those bitter memories you were telling us about from the time of your parents' divorce? [What do you think?]" However, it is not unusual for such interpretations to shift down into the lower-right quadrant where they represent a controlling posture: "You may not have thought of this, but it is clear to me that your recurrent patterns of leaving your partners on short notice represent a childlike avoidance of facing issues. [Please give some thought to what I know is wrong with you.]" Critical comments that portray a judgmental and critical attitude that may trigger defensiveness may also be inserted under the guise of interpretation: "It seems that you have again failed to appreciate how you become trapped in these self-destructive relationships [stupid]."

Thus, both clarification and confrontational interventions may have the same interactional process message. However, confrontation techniques are more liable to contain alternative or mixed process messages that may be less therapeutic in nature. There is some advantage therefore to considering carefully which method to use. If in doubt, the clarification approach has less potential for misuse. Of course, there is a middle ground in which clarification techniques are used to direct attention to a particular issue in a manner that is essentially interpretive: "You said earlier that you couldn't stand your father, now you are feeling quite angry with Dan. Could you clarify for me how you see the two of them as being alike? [Go ahead and make your own linking interpretation.]"

Another useful idea for group use is borrowed from the family therapy literature. This consists of efforts to elicit differential perceptions and reactions among the participants. This may be done by having various members describe what they saw happening or what they thought a particular incident or behavior might mean. This elicits a variety of opinions that can then be compared and contrasted. Ranking questions are also a powerful way of stimulating thoughtful exchanges, for example, "Who in the group do you think would be most critical of you if you said that?" These techniques tease out differences that stimulate intense involvement and the need to individuate opinions. Thus, they promote an interactive environment in which individual positions and opinions are sought and held as important.

Timing of Interventions

The question of timing is crucial to effective interventions. The most accurate and eloquent interpretation given at the wrong time will be wasted. The usual problem is making an intervention too early. Perhaps with some anxiety that something needs to be said, the therapist will move in too quickly with a lengthy statement that takes the pressure off the group for developing its own initiative. A good rule of thumb is that an interpretation should be made just before the individual is about ready to put it into words anyway. If that is the case, then sometimes a simple stimulus question will enable members to develop their own interpretative thought. An approach that encourages patients to reach their own conclusions provides an autonomy-developing style that can be transferred to outside situations. A good therapeutic outcome is one where patients can think back on therapy as a process by which they learned to understand their problems with the encouragement of the therapist. This point is particularly relevant to group therapy, in which any given member has the advantage of receiving reflective or interpretative statements from anyone in the group. By holding back, the leader leaves the field open for helpful statements from other members, thus promoting the therapeutic factor of altruism.

Once an interpretation has been made, it is important to carefully monitor whether the result was further opening up and exploration or a state of greater defensiveness and withdrawal. This usually occurs within the next few minutes. It will indicate to the therapist the accuracy of the timing judgment.

Level of Interpretation

The approach to group psychotherapy described in this book has emphasized the use of group therapeutic factors and interpersonal learning factors. A somewhat different perspective is provided by psychoanalytically trained group therapists. They are more inclined to emphasize internal mental connections and to view the central change-inducing mechanism in terms of the interpretive process. Technically, a higher proportion of interventions will deal with unconscious transferential material, and the role of the therapist is more central to the group task. Much of the recent psychoanalytic group therapy literature describes the management of patients with narcissistic or borderline character pathology.

The first important concept is the idea of blocked responses that emerge in distorted or inappropriate ways, usually with a high level of affect. These "split-off" parts of relationship qualities may then be projected onto individuals in the group, resulting in serious misinterpretations and unstable, shifting reactions. Strong use of denial mechanisms may accompany these processes. The relationship to the therapist is seen as a particularly important area to understand. It is representative of parental/authority issues, and the personal responses experienced by the therapist may offer important clues to the nature of the distortions being projected by the patient. The group context itself has been described in terms of the group representing a maternal entity, the group as mother. This may be idealized by the patient as the source of endless gratification, or feared as threatening engulfment. The group context, with its quality of normative expectations, may exacerbate fears of being shamed, fears that may resonate with childhood memories.

From a therapeutic standpoint, the group has been characterized as a "holding environment" that serves to contain the highly charged split-off reactions until they can be synthesized into a more stable sense of self-identity. The acceptance and positive mirroring of a cohesive group are seen as important factors in this process, an expression of empathy to the individual's needs, if not to the behaviors (66).

There is a spectrum of opinion regarding the question of which level of conceptualization is most effective. Use of group-level interpretations as the only approach, as used in Tavistock groups, has already been discouraged because the level of abstraction makes it difficult for the members to use the material effectively. There is meager research evidence regarding the differential value of addressing interpersonal transactions or intrapsychic mechanisms. There is reasonable support for the importance of a consistent focus on a central theme, however defined. In actual practice, most practitioners use a mixture of interpretive positions. In Chapter 10, the use of the "two triangles" to conceptualize important interpersonal dimensions is derived from analytic ideas transformed into interpersonal language. There tends to be greater agreement between observers about what is going on when interpersonal language is used. Throughout this book, the admonition of the integrationists to use "plain English" has been generally followed. This is a good rule for the clinician as well. Better an accurate description than a fuzzy theoretical concept.

Preventing Negative Effects

No therapist wants to do harm. However, many patients terminate their group experience before they have had a chance to benefit from it. Others report, even years later, that they experienced their therapy as personally damaging. This is usually related to a critical incident that involves self-esteem issues leading to a lasting effect of demoralization or unresolved anger.

The percentage of premature terminators from therapy groups ranges from 10% to as high as 50%. The majority of these dropouts occur within the first six sessions. This suggests that selection, composition, and entry factors are responsible. Unplanned termination later in a group's life usually involves either a specific upsetting incident or resistance to addressing specific problem areas. An additional unfortunate effect for both dropouts and casualties is that they may be discouraged from seeking further professional help in the future.

The remainder of this chapter pulls together issues that have been touched on elsewhere in the book representing errors of judgment or dangerous situations that predispose to negative effects. This checklist of predisposing or precipitating factors is devoted to the ancient nostrum *primum non nocere*, "above all do no harm" (67).

Errors of Selection and Composition

Some casualties are set up through errors of clinical judgment made before the group begins. This involves questions of assessment and group composition described in Chapters 6 and 7. Patients with a marked paranoid style may set themselves up for a negative experience. The stimulation of the group environment usually exacerbates such qualities, which in turn produces a negative reaction from other members. Thus, both the group and the individual suffer. Similarly, patients who use extremely brittle denial may be unable to use group interaction constructively and antagonize the group. Major schizoid traits may be interpreted by the other members as resistance or implied criticism, and the schizoid patient may find himself or herself in a scapegoated position that exacerbates preexisting doubts about social competency. A serious misalignment of expectations about therapy will create problems and may on occasion result in the individual eliciting a rejecting response from group members that produces a harmful effect.

Developmental Stage

Circumstances that are likely to increase the risk of negative effects can be predicted on the basis of group development. The following issues are presented in the sequential order in which they might appear in a group.

1. *Not belonging.* In the early sessions, the group must develop cohesion. Central to this is a sense of belongingness. If a member actively experiences being outside of the group culture, not belonging, this has the potential for a powerful negative effect. The

therapist has a specific responsibility to monitor for this sort of development. The issue must be addressed promptly.

2. *Excessive self-disclosure.* The revelation of highly charged factual material, such as incestuous experiences, homosexuality, or violent crimes, can be harmful if it is presented before the development of a strong supportive atmosphere. The group may find it overwhelming and, in order to preserve an emerging sense of cohesion, may isolate or attack the individual.

3. *Early conflict.* Similarly, the early eruption of significant conflict before the group has become consolidated is likely to be poorly tolerated and lead to early dropouts. This is often found in groups that fail to develop a sense of cohesion.

4. *Attack or rejection.* The confrontational process of the differentiation stage becomes dangerous when there is a perception that it is driven by the intent to harm, disgrace, or reject the recipient. The therapist must be on guard for such qualities.

5. *Scapegoating.* This group phenomenon can be particularly damaging because the individual is left alone to face the entire group. An intense and unresolved process of scapegoating entails serious risk for a negative effect and premature termination.

6. *Lack of response from others.* Many critical incidents are characterized by heightened levels of affect. Because such intensity may be threatening to the group members, a powerfully felt statement may be met with silence. Being left "up in the air" with no response can be a devastating experience. It may be interpreted as a rejection of the individual or a condemnation of the subject matter. In states of high emotion, there is more susceptibility to distorted interpretations, so the therapist may need to intervene to bring the group back to the issue so that the affective dimension can be diffused. Otherwise, the involved individual may resolve never again to risk so much.

There is the added danger that a person may leave a session having misinterpreted the meaning of the group's response, convinced of his or her own stupidity or worthlessness, and perhaps with thoughts of self-destructive behavior. It is appropriate for the therapist to ask a member to stay after the session so that an assessment of clinical safety can be made.

7. *Sexual relationships between members.* The emergence of overt sexual behavior between group members is always a serious matter. This is not because of issues of morality, though that may

be a consideration. An ongoing intimate relationship between two group members largely precludes their effective use of the group. They will have secrets to be kept from the group and will have difficulty maintaining a therapeutic attitude regarding their own relationship. A therapy group is not real life, it is a simulation, and when that distinction is lost, the learning potential drops. It is incumbent on the therapist to resolve the situation. This usually involves meeting with the involved members outside of group and reaching a decision about who should terminate from this particular therapy group.

   Some such episodes involve irresponsible actions by members who take advantage of the naïveté or distress of others. Unfortunately, those who are victimized often have had similar experiences before entering the group and view this as a further demonstration of their own vulnerability and inability to master their environment. Thus, the experiences may exacerbate an already tarnished sense of self-esteem.

8. *Termination.*   The stress of termination, if not handled appropriately, may result in a panicky sense of abandonment or dissatisfaction. This may interfere with a constructive internalization of the group experience. Sometimes under the stress of termination, compensatory and destructive decisions may be made such as an impulsive involvement in other relationships or an increase in suicidal thoughts. All of this underlines the need to deal persistently with termination issues. The therapist's reluctance to deal with separation may contribute to these problems.

Leadership Style

Excessive confrontation.   An aggressively confrontational style is often associated with charismatic qualities that demand followership. The danger of this style lies in the possibility of leading some members into levels of self-disclosure or risk taking that they are not able to tolerate. They may leave a session only to recognize that they have gone far beyond the bounds they consider appropriate, regret this in a shameful or fearful manner, and never return. Over time, the memory of the event increasingly takes on the qualities of an attack in which they were the helpless victims. This may result in an enduring sense of having been violated, of vulnerability, and of unwillingness to trust other therapeutic situations.

Distant and aloof therapists. Such therapists fail to provide adequate guidance or direction for the group and commonly experience higher numbers of dropouts as the group does not become engaged. However, these therapeutic "sins of omission" are less likely to be associated with specific harmful effects.

Attacks and criticism. There is little room for the direct expression of hostility, anger, or aggression in psychotherapy. Professionals with a significant tendency to blame, criticize, or ridicule their patients have a higher rate of negative effects. "I can't help that, it's their fault," they would say. Such professionals are best to work in other areas.

Summary

This chapter has looked in more detail at the relationship between the therapist and the group. Issues related to neutrality and intervention style are closely connected to the person of the therapist. For this reason, an experiential component in the training for group psychotherapy is important. The group situation contains the potential for harm. Typical risky situations are outlined. The therapist must be prepared to actively manage these when they arise.

Professional Practice

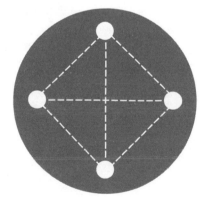

CHAPTER 14

Group Programs

Group programs are found in all aspects of the mental health service delivery system. They are particularly common in settings associated with hospitals, mental health centers, and multispecialty clinics. In such larger systems, the steady flow of patients facilitates the organization of therapy groups. This includes the possibility of specialty groups for targeted populations. This chapter will address some of the common issues involved in setting up group therapy programs in a diversity of settings.

Evidence for Change

Effectiveness of Group Psychotherapy

Recent literature reviews indicate that psychotherapy is generally quite effective. Meta-analyses of outcome studies have yielded positive findings with an effect size in the range of .85, indicating that the average treated person is better off than 80% of the untreated sample. Group psychotherapy by itself is indicated in circumstances that are clearly reactions to specific stress or to recurrent patterns of interpersonal difficulties. These factors are often combined. Psychotic symptoms such as hallucinations, delusions, and melancholia require psychopharmacologic management; however, numerous studies suggest that the addition of a psychotherapeutic component to the pharmacologic treatment regimen enhances outcome results. The psychotherapy may directly complement the action of medication, producing a higher overall rate of response. Improved personal adjustment may reduce the exposure to stressful precipitating events. Finally, a good working alliance will improve compliance with medication regimens (68).

The situation is less clear in the large number of patients presenting with mixed symptoms of anxiety and depression, often in the context of unfortunate relationship situations. Some authors suggest that these patients represent examples of less extreme affective illness. Others understand them as reflective of maladaptive learned interpersonal behavior. Many seem to indicate a vicious circle in which poor relationships lead to unhappiness, and this demoralized and self-critical condition contributes to less effective coping. In such situations, antidepressant medications are less specifically effective and minor tranquilizers usually make things worse. Psychotherapy may help general adaptation, but often does not result in total relief of symptoms. In this gray area of unhappy and dysfunctional people, the relative contributions of talking and pills require further investigation. In particular, studies looking for more specific indicators of response are needed, so that there can be greater precision in fitting the patient with the most appropriate treatment modality (69).

Few studies have directly compared individual therapy with group therapy. Some of the better comparative studies are reviewed in the Source Notes. Generally speaking, there appears to be minimal difference in therapeutic outcome between the two modalities. There is a suggestion that the premature termination rate from group therapy may be less than from individual therapy. The more important issue is not whether a particular approach is "better" than another, but rather which patients are most suited to which modality (70).

A related aspect is the degree of patient satisfaction from different types of psychotherapy. In a recent study, patients were randomly assigned to brief individual or group psychotherapy. The group patients improved as much as those in individual therapy, but they expressed less satisfaction with the treatment. Despite this, the dropout rate was no larger in the group component. If groups are to be widely used in an outpatient clinic program, then specific efforts must be taken to prepare patients to alter their attitudes toward the idea of group therapy. This underlines the need for systematic pretherapy preparation as a means to combat premature termination and enhance motivation (71).

The outcome literature provides justification for greater use of

group psychotherapy approaches. Groups appear to offer equal therapeutic outcome with greater efficiency. It is not unreasonable to suggest that group therapy be regarded as the therapeutic modality of
choice unless family approaches are indicated. Individual therapy beyond an initial assessment phase should be carefully reviewed for its
appropriateness. These ideas are of particular interest as financial
restraints on the health-care dollar are increasing. This position is not
a popular one. Most clinicians have not been well trained in the theory
and practice of group psychotherapy and may therefore regard it as a
secondary treatment modality. To suggest that it ranks as a full equal
with the traditional hour of individual therapy seems heretical. The
evidence suggests otherwise.

Group therapy offers unique advantages. The supportive cluster
of therapeutic factors tends to be more intense in groups than in
individual therapy. In particular, universalization and altruism have
more impact. Groups offer a broader array of opportunities for modeling and vicarious learning. Above all, group cohesiveness and acceptance have quite a different quality of "normalization" than the therapeutic alliance in individual therapy. Similarly, the process of
psychological learning is conducted in a different fashion. In groups,
there is an opportunity for multiple stimulus relationships. Patients
can see themselves in others and therefore view their own behavior
more objectively. Feedback from group members is often more direct
and to the point than in individual sessions. The process of risk taking
in groups results in ideas that are more easily applied to outside
circumstances. Overall, group psychotherapy is conducted in a social
atmosphere that is closer to normal life circumstances, and transfer of
learning is therefore enhanced.

Time and Clinical Change

The idea of setting a specific time limit to a course of psychotherapy may seem like a simple strategy, but in practice, theory and
technique vary considerably. Several large surveys of the practice of
outpatient psychotherapy reveal that attendance figures in all service
systems show a steeply falling distribution curve. As Figure 14-1
reveals, in most outpatient programs, about two-thirds of the patients
are seen for 6 sessions or less, and less than 10% attend for more than
25 sessions (72).

Interpretation of this attrition curve raises important issues. If the
curve falls too quickly, it suggests that the service is failing to live up

Percent

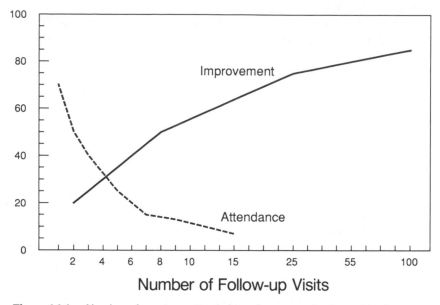

Figure 14-1. Number of sessions attended in a large sample of psychiatric outpatient clinics and the rate of symptomatic improvement. Both curves are based on large, but not identical, samples.

to its own expectations. A larger than anticipated number of patients are being seen for very brief contact in comparison to those who are being seen for longer care. Intake screening and the entry process may need to be reviewed. Conversely, if the right-hand side of the curve is proportionately too high, it suggests that the service is overburdened with longer-term cases and is not providing optimal treatment for the greatest number of patients admitted to it. Some system of caseload management triggered by length of treatment might be helpful. Service utilization figures such as these are a useful starting point when reviewing an outpatient clinic. They have direct relevance to the sorts of programs that would be most effective in meeting the needs of the population served.

A related question is whether longer-term treatment has greater change effects than shorter-term treatment. Is there some break point where maximum effect is achieved? Recent reviews of a large number of outcome studies have plotted improvement rates as a function of time. Quite consistently in outpatient samples, approximately 50% of patients showed significant improvement by the 8th session, and 75%

by the 26th session (see Figure 14-1). Patients engaged in longer-term treatment showed the same early improvement in symptoms as those in brief therapy. These results apply whether the outcome data are obtained from the patients themselves, from the therapist, or from objective ratings. In light of these figures, it would be reasonable to consider a careful clinical review of those patients who have not shown measurable improvement by the 26th session (73).

In the clinical literature, the range of sessions for patients in crisis is usually about 6 sessions and for brief individual therapy is from 12 to 25 sessions. These numbers seem quite in keeping with the empirical data just reviewed. If one assumes that clinical change is a function of therapeutic exposure plus time to adapt, then it could be argued that the session range might be extended somewhat for group therapy while still adhering to the idea of a definite time limit. Indeed, it is usual in the group literature to see results of time-limited groups running from 8 to about 40 sessions. If one calculates on the basis of groups with eight members, then forty 90-minute sessions comes out to about 8 hours per member. Of course, in groups there is the opportunity for vicarious learning throughout the session so that the exposure time is underestimated. Therefore, the "dose" of psychotherapy is in the same range as that found in the individual therapy literature.

Planning for Group Programs

Planning for group programs must involve administrative representatives at an early stage. This forces the clinicians involved to articulate the goals, target populations, and management strategies they are considering. If this is done in a collaborative fashion, there is less chance that groups will be designed for which there is insufficient patient flow. Administrative support can make it easier to get referrals, to find space resources, and to avoid schedule conflicts. Because groups offer more efficient use of staff time, they are usually welcomed by program planners. This may not be the best reason to run groups, but it is a good rationale for mobilizing support for group program development.

The clinician is in a position to judge whether the desired goals can be reasonably addressed in the time frame being considered. Programs may develop module patterns of 8-, 12-, or 20-session packages. For some purposes, these are very suitable, and the time frame forces intense and focused work. If there is a mismatch between time and the likelihood of change, however, such arrangements may promote therapeutic nihilism or offer an invitation for avoidance of sustained work. Six months of uninterrupted therapy may have a greater effect than two 12-session blocks with a changed group membership.

Just as the group member functions within the context of the group system, so the group itself operates as part of a larger service delivery system. It is useful to begin the planning process with a careful look at this larger system. This might include a review of service attendance data as mentioned above, as well as a breakdown by large diagnostic categories. How many patients need longer-term supportive approaches that could be provided more effectively, not just more efficiently, in a group format? Could the services of clinic psychiatrists be used more efficiently if they were to participate in full or in part in groups in which regular review of medications is indicated? Would the creation of groups provide an opportunity for suitable patients to receive more intensive psychotherapy than is otherwise available because of service-load constraints? Could some staff begin a process of specialization, for example, in groups for treatment of adolescent problems, or addictive problems, or eating disorder problems? This often has a spin-off effect of increasing staff morale. The idea of implementing group programs may meet with staff resistance because it is seen only as a way to churn more patients through the system. Staff need to know that allowance will be made for the extra energy needed for running groups, as well as some system of in-house supervision or training. The planning exercise will be more effective if it includes opportunities for input at all levels.

Part of the planning exercise is to assess the group expertise within the professional staff. It is common to encounter the attitude that group therapy is appropriately designated to the least qualified staff. This seems to be based on some notion that less skill is required in treating several patients than in treating one. As indicated throughout this book, an understanding of the group system and the skills appropriate thereto is superimposed on a basic grounding in assessing and treating the individual. Part of the misrepresentation of groups is through the notion that the group therapist has less responsibility because "the patients treat themselves." Although it is true that an important aspect of group therapy is the opportunity for member-to-member interactions, groups have considerable potential for harm or at the very least for avoidance. The group therapist's responsibility spans a broader ground than in individual work, because not only the therapist can do harm, so can the rest of the group.

Scheduling of Groups

Weekly outpatient groups, the most common format, generally need several sessions to develop good levels of cohesion. At that point, stage 2 issues of conflict begin to emerge. It is worth planning, therefore, to begin a group with the clear prospect of at least 6–8 sessions before the likelihood of a significant interruption. It is even better to think of 12 uninterrupted sessions. There is some advantage to thinking in seasonal terms. This is particularly compatible with the time-limited approach. A group beginning in September can have about 12 sessions before the New Year's interruption. Similarly, groups beginning in January can count on a lengthy interruption-free introductory period. It is important that all members attend all early sessions. This necessitates a careful review with potential group members as to the practicalities of the next 6–8 weeks. Business trips, vacations, or exams can become convenient rationales for lack of enthusiasm in the treatment process.

Similar consideration should be given to the time the group meets. If it appears that a particular member might have to miss every second or fourth session because of unnegotiable time conflicts, then that person needs another type of therapy. The patient should be supportively informed of this and alternative arrangements made. As potential members of a group are being collected, it is worth delaying the beginning of the group somewhat if it means that early interruptions can be avoided.

Similar care should be given to deciding whether group membership is to be considered open. One advantage of time-limited groups is the opportunity for the group to begin, mature, and end together. This encourages a systematic focus on the issues relevant to each stage in a context in which all the members can appreciate the same issues. I strongly recommend that time-limited groups be closed. If for unpredictable reasons new members must be added, then this should be done with some consideration to the current thematic material. In particular, an assessment should be made as to the penetration of conflict issues within the group. New members should be added in advance of these or after they are under reasonable cognitive control. The addition of new members will always induce group regression. The safest time for the addition of new members is after the group has matured into a functional, cohesive state.

There is a danger that new members will be scapegoated as the parties responsible for the group's need to go through engagement issues once again. For that reason, it is a good general policy to add new members in pairs. This builds in a peer relationship for the newcomers that provides some buffering against the introduction stresses. There are often problems when a large number of group members are replaced at once, for example, if four new members are added to the remaining four from an ongoing group. New versus old subgroups tend to arise that may be very resistant to melding.

Questions of attendance and membership address external boundary issues that must not be handled casually. Sometimes new group therapists are reluctant to be specific about such matters because they fear they might lose a potential member. It is much better to drop a member before the group begins than for the group to suffer the demoralizing effects of early dropouts. By careful attention to organizational details, the therapist is creating a "frame" for the group experience, within which meaningful use can be made of each member's participation.

In Chapter 16, the importance of prompt and systematic record keeping is discussed. When a group is being set up, time should be allowed for this activity. Most groups are scheduled to run for 75–90 minutes. This is enough time to allow reasonable opportunities for participation by all members. Groups that are largely supportive in nature or that deal with patients with low attention spans may be shorter, say 45–60 minutes. The therapist should add a minimum of one half hour of open time around that allowed for the group itself. Ten to 15 minutes in advance to review the records of the preceding session, to consider an agenda of important issues for this session, and to get back into the group atmosphere is time well spent. For an experienced therapist, 15 or 20 minutes is required at the end of a group to document the session and spend a few minutes pondering the important issues as an aide-mémoire for review before the next session. For more extensive postgroup discussion, particularly in the case of new therapists or when cotherapy is used, additional time is required. These time issues should be part of the basic planning structure of the group and not something considered to be optional or squeezed in between other clinical activities.

Cotherapy Issues

Many group therapy programs encourage the use of cotherapists. Queries as to the reason for this are usually met with surprise that the practice would even be questioned. However, there are significant potential problems as well as advantages to be considered (74).

The addition of a cotherapist to a small group increases the interactional possibilities. Role functions may be differentially shared. One therapist can monitor group reactions when the other is more intensely involved. The observing therapist can then help to manage the interaction between the group and that partner. However, such functions are extremely delicate. Such a situation is loaded with potential for competitive interactions between therapists, for perceived criticisms, and so on. Serious cotherapy work is for advanced therapists who enjoy a close working relationship.

Seeing such an experienced and compatible cotherapy pair at work can be a delight. But all too often, the cotherapy relationship is used as a means of avoiding issues. Rather than a strategy of strength, it can become a strategy of weakness. Comments such as, "I was going to take that up, but I thought you were working on something else," offer a rationale for therapist passivity. Therapist challenge is an important process in most therapy groups. With two therapists to confront, members may be reluctant to move into this sensitive area. Under the guise of assisting such work, it is not uncommon for cotherapists in fact to deflect or dampen the process of therapist challenge.

Sometimes cotherapy is used because the therapists, often junior staff members, are both inadequately trained—two half-trained therapists equal one fully trained one? Such a model combines the worst of both worlds. Not only are the therapists faced with the complexity of running a group, but they must also deal with complications of the cotherapy relationship and its impact on the group. To make matters worse, sometimes such pairing is accompanied by a rotation system so that the pairs are always changing. A possible exception to these pessimistic comments is inpatient ward groups in which several staff members may be involved, often in accordance with rotation schedules. In such groups, there is greater emphasis on the group culture and less on leader-member interaction. The group is an extension from the general ward milieu. Such groups are discussed in more detail later in this chapter.

A case can be made for the use of solo therapists as the norm, with special circumstances justifying cotherapy. With a single therapist, there is one person with a clear mandate of responsibility. That person has the opportunity to pursue a consistent path of tracking group themes and planning therapeutic strategies. When cotherapy is used, special attention must be focused on the cotherapy partnership. It creates a therapist subsystem that will be the subject of close scrutiny by the members. The therapists must be continuously aware of the state of their own interaction as well as that of the group members. This complexity increases the likelihood of issues being missed or not addressed because of uncertainty about responsibility. Cotherapists must be sure to systematically debrief after sessions, and the question of their relationship in the group must be constantly reviewed.

Some types of groups might benefit from cotherapy pairs. For example, the presence of a male and female therapist may offer parental imagery that is helpful for adolescent groups. Similarly, a mixed-gender cotherapy pair may be useful for patients with eating disorders in whom gender-related issues must be addressed. Couples groups should offer a model of a cotherapy relationship that facilitates identification with gender roles. Note that in all of these examples, it is the quality of the cotherapist relationship that confers the added benefit.

The cotherapy model can be useful for training purposes. One version of this is to pair a trainee with an experienced therapist. This has the advantage of providing a modeling experience and an opportunity for the junior trainee to experience group events without feeling total responsibility for managing them. There is also the opportunity for a detailed review of the sessions to integrate theory and clinical intervention style. In some situations, two trainees will colead a group. Such circumstances need to be carefully supervised, preferably with observation or videotaping techniques. Either of these training experiences needs to be complemented at some point with an opportunity for the trainee to run groups alone under supervision.

When a decision is made to utilize cotherapy, care should be taken in the pair selection process. It is important that a cotherapy dyad demonstrate respectful adult interaction. A sense of rapport and goodwill and a comfortableness between the two is essential. A marked difference in dominance, or a substantial quality of competition may be damaging to a group. It is possible for the group to become polarized around attachment to each leader. Although cotherapists will always have some differences in style, group members may become confused if there is a marked variation in technique. Cotherapists must be able to accommodate and tolerate differences without slipping into self-justifying positions.

A particular set of cotherapy issues arises when the two leaders are of opposite sex. In some ways, this is the preferred arrangement because it provides a model of interaction and of transference potential that may be very helpful for group members struggling with gender-related interpersonal issues. There are inherent stresses related to traditional gender role expectations that need to be taken into account. Opposite-sex cotherapists rapidly activate parental images for the members. These are often heavily loaded identifications and may result in skewed perceptions about therapist behavior. Certainly, the nature of the cotherapist relationship will be closely watched and will be the source of much fantasy material. This provides rich opportunities for psychotherapeutic work, but the therapists must be prepared to tackle such material comfortably and directly.

Cotherapy issues usually occur in the context of larger systems where there are junior staff and trainees who need to be accommodated. The choice of cotherapy should be made only after careful consideration and with suitable supervision safeguards. Staff who thought they were committed to the cotherapy model often experience a sense of exhilaration and professional growth once they begin to run groups alone.

Combining Therapies

There are many possible combinations of therapies. In each case, specific boundary issues may occur. It is useful, sometimes crucial, that these sorts of boundary dilemmas be considered in any of the complex situations that can arise in daily practice. Some mechanism should be in place for regular interchange of information among those providing different approaches to the patient. This fundamental guideline applies to all of the examples discussed below.

Medication Checks

A common occurrence is for a patient in group psychotherapy to also be seeing a referring psychiatrist at less frequent intervals for review of medication. This situation offers golden opportunities for the patient to work one against the other. For example, a group may be encouraging a patient to address important personal issues that are being enacted with other group members, a process producing an increase in anxiety. The patient then visits the psychiatrist for the ostensible purpose of having medications reviewed. Group events are misrepresented or not mentioned at all, and the patient comes away with the recommendation to increase medications and miss a few sessions until feeling better. A more suitable format for conducting supportive follow-up groups is found later in this chapter.

Multiple Groups

It is not uncommon to find a patient enrolled in several groups simultaneously. Such situations commonly occur in inpatient units, day hospitals, or other intensive treatment settings. These groups often go under interesting names such as feelings groups, life-style groups, social skills groups, assertiveness groups, etc. In one program, the label "feelings group" was applied because nonphysicians were not supposed to do real therapy, but they could talk about feelings!

There is nothing necessarily wrong with several approaches. Sometimes diversity can stimulate creative opportunities. But very often, the various types of groups are developed because of the particular interest of a staff member or an administrative decision that such and such a program must be started because the hospital across town has one. Careful thought should be given to the advantages to the patient of being in the same group more frequently rather than bouncing around among a variety of different therapists and approaches. Assertiveness issues can be reasonably approached in a general group setting. Application to outside social circumstances certainly needs to be addressed in most group work. And of course, those notorious feelings flow through all of the groups. A particularly virulent form of group proliferation results from the determination of each professional discipline to have its own program, which then runs in subtle competition with the others. The responsible clinician must seriously address the question of what each modality adds to justify the extra therapeutic experience.

Concurrent Individual and Group Therapy

A particular example of concurrent therapy is the use of individual and group treatment scheduled on a regular basis as a specific therapeutic strategy. This is more common in large metropolitan areas where there is an abundance of therapeutic resources. *Combined therapy* refers to individual and group therapy provided by the same therapist. The term *conjoint therapy* is used to describe concurrent therapy by two different therapists. Theoretically, the individual context offers an opportunity to explore the emotional reactions of personal history at more length and to develop insight concerning the conflictual issues inherent in them. The group context is particularly effective for applying new behaviors and receiving feedback concerning them. Relationships with a variety of people can be explored, giving greater opportunity for identifying interpersonal distortions. These working-through processes are reinforced by the greater independence promoted by the group context.

There is a serious potential of destructive competition between the two approaches. The patient may feel that the individual setting is the "real therapy" and use it to drain off tension from group work. On the other hand, individual sessions may be used to rehash group events, thus interfering with productive individual work. In both directions, the information provided by the patient may not be complete or may be significantly distorted. The individual therapist or the group may react with astonishment, even outrage, to what is presumed to be going on. Such experiences are ideally suited for enhancing individual resistance.

Because of these predictable problems, the decision to engage in concurrent therapy must be carefully considered. The involvement of two different therapists increases the problems. When two therapists are involved, particular attention must be paid to the ground rules concerning communication between them. The goal is to build in regular communication so that the sorts of difficulties mentioned above can be prevented. This is easiest when the two modalities are being provided in the same clinical setting or between colleagues who know each other well.

Issues of confidentiality pose a particular problem. With formal combined therapy, the safest approach is to insist that information provided in the individual context is in fact group information and vice versa. Awkward situations may arise in the group around who is going to introduce the subject matter, but this is preferable to maintaining secrets between the two settings. Prior agreement about this issue promotes a clearer understanding that the purpose of the individual component is to amplify and clarify therapeutic events, not to function as a totally separate treatment system. The decision to share information is clearly one that must be made in the light of clinical judgment. The implementation of these ideas is obviously easier if the same therapist is involved in both modalities. Similar principles apply to other concurrent treatment situations. The question of between-session phone calls or emergencies is discussed in the next chapter. In all of the above situations, the ground rules of confidentiality must be very clear (75).

Sequential Therapies

The decision to shift to group therapy after a period of individual work is fraught with problems. The patient will almost always view this as a demotion if not outright abandonment. When such a change is a possibility, it should be introduced at an early point in individual therapy and kept in the conversation as a recurring theme. The individual work can be characterized as a time of preparation for the group. The point of change may represent a phase shift, often from crisis intervention to ongoing psychotherapy. Consideration should be given to making this transition quite explicit with a short break in therapy and transfer to another therapist. The transition from well-established individual therapy to group therapy with another therapist is particularly hazardous. A large number of dropouts can be anticipated without very careful preparation.

Conversely, a shift from group to individual therapy may also be considered. This has fewer intrinsic problems of implementation. The principal concern in this situation has to do with the motivation for the change. It may represent a capitulation to patient resistance in the group. If so, the individual sessions are also unlikely to be productive. In general, groups are more effective in challenging resistances than individual therapists, so the result is likely to be an implicit pact that things will not be stirred up. This may be quite appropriate, but the decision should be made with a clear mind.

One sequential model suggests that therapy be started with individual therapy, and then continued in group therapy with the same therapist. This gives the therapist a useful perspective on how the patient reacts in two quite different settings. The therapist has first-hand knowledge of both and is in a better position to use each for its intended purpose. The transition between modalities is a critical time. Many patients experience considerable difficulty in giving up the one-to-one relationship with the therapist, and premature terminations are a danger.

Inpatient Groups

Inpatient groups face many unique difficulties. Patient turnover is rapid, the level of patient pathology is high, motivation may be low, and the mix of problems is continually fluctuating. Investigations and treatments are in progress simultaneously, often producing scheduling problems. Psychotropic medications may interfere with cognitive functioning. There are many different professionals involved in patient care. These problems are becoming increasingly evident as the average length of stay on inpatient units drops. In the face of all of this, groups remain a important feature of the inpatient milieu. Patients regularly report that they have received considerable help from the ward group experience (76).

Various strategies have been devised to make the most of this difficult situation. It should be clearly recognized that the group component to inpatient care is only one part of treatment. Other treatments will deal with other things. The goals for inpatient groups need to be limited to realistic levels. Groups can be of most help by focusing on interpersonal behavior with an educational orientation. The core group experience has been described as one of learning to think therapeutically.

Patients should be selected to attend group only if they can to some extent stay seated and attend to the process. Most patients experiencing acute psychotic states or major depressions can do so. Mute, incoherent, or extremely labile patients are inappropriate. Acute mania is a contraindication until the patient begins to settle. One of the therapists should spend a few minutes with patients before they begin the group to provide a fast orientation. This might consist of a brief description of when the group meets and what the main goals are. Basic ground rules concerning attendance, participation, and confidentiality are reviewed. Ward groups are best limited to 60 minutes. Even shorter groups are indicated for patients with significant cognitive dysfunction. The ability to maintain attention will deteriorate quickly under the interactional demands of a group setting.

It is most common to divide patients into groups based on a two-level system of interactional capacity. One group contains patients suffering from psychotic experiences including the effects of organic impairment, and the other is composed of those patients who are able to talk more actively regarding interpersonal matters. There will always be a gray area between these two categories that can be used to create two roughly equally sized groups at any one point in time. Some programs restrict entry into ward groups to Mondays, thus achieving some degree of membership stability for at least a week. Because the patients are actually interacting throughout the day, such arrangements may allow the development of more advanced group work.

Inpatient groups can be conceptualized as remaining forever in stage 1. They are continually rebeginning and struggling to consolidate the group's external boundary. Therapeutic factors from the supportive cluster should be mobilized: acceptance, hope, universality, and altruism. A positive orientation should be encouraged, and the group purposefully discouraged from getting into the leader challenges of stage 2. There is seldom enough time or group stability to hope to get through such material satisfactorily. The content focus is maintained stringently on the circumstances that led to hospitalization, coping with current symptoms, and preparing for discharge. This includes information about medications and the role of stress in precipitating symptoms. Reference to discharge planning is begun immediately, including ideas about how to stay out of the hospital. The emphasis is on coping with current problems, not curing symptoms. Therapists will find useful ideas from the crisis intervention literature. This is focused on the tasks of mobilization of affect, clarification of the issues and circumstances, and then a problem-solving review of alternative strategies (77).

This approach has major implications for therapeutic technique. The therapist must be active, positive, and supportive—in control of the group. The focus of the group is on information more than affect. Specific attention is paid to the circumstances of admission. An educational component can be introduced at any time and applied to the particular circumstances of each member. Patients are encouraged to think about their treatment from a therapeutic standpoint. What clues can they use to identify problems early? How can they seek help before the need for hospitalization arises? What are the effects and side effects of the medication they are taking? Details of past history and dynamic interpretations are out of place. Sanction and support are given for patients talking among themselves between sessions, something they will be doing anyway. This focus will sensitize patients to treatment issues and increase their motivation to comply with outpatient arrangements. Therapists who are familiar with the more orderly pace and greater psychological mindedness of outpatient groups may regard inpatient work as superficial and ineffective. However, to lead an inpatient group with the mind-set of achieving great psychological insight is not only frustrating, it is not in the best interest of the patients.

Ward groups do not exist in a vacuum, but actively reflect ward issues. On short-stay wards, this usually involves ward crises. For patients on longer-stay wards, the opportunity to participate in frequent sessions may result in very intensive therapeutic work. Complex management issues may emerge, particularly involving patients who are able to split staff reactions. Higher-functioning ward groups provide an opportunity to focus on the importance of a dynamic orientation in understanding the person who also happens to have a psychiatric illness.

Many units have regular community meetings of all patients and most staff members. The large number of participants means that the meeting cannot function as a therapy group. A more suitable structure is that of a town hall meeting with a chairperson and an agenda. The presence of this structure paradoxically results in greater freedom to participate because there is not the expectation that attention will be focused on every phrase. Topics can include planning of ward activities, management of the problems of living together, specific ward incidents, and information about procedures, meetings, and so on. Such meetings can be quite helpful in maintaining a sense of ward tradition and in mediating problems before they become too highly charged.

Supportive Follow-up Groups

A major challenge to the mental health care delivery system is the provision of adequate programs for patients with major psychiatric illness requiring long-term follow-up. This particularly concerns patients with schizophrenia and the more severe bipolar affective disorders. This section is specifically titled "supportive groups" rather than "medication groups" because the task for these programs goes well beyond simple medication review. Long-term follow-up is effectively, perhaps preferentially, provided through group programs. Patients falling into these diagnostic categories have many common issues. The use of long-term medication produces many problems. Support is needed in adapting to and managing the inevitable side effects. Most of these patients have significant problems in daily living both in terms of residential placements and employment. Many programs have found it useful to encourage, rather than discourage, extragroup socializing. In this way, closer attention can be paid to the realities of daily life and how they can be addressed.

There are many ways for organizing supportive follow-up groups. All of them must deal with the fact that attendance is expected to be both long-term and episodic and that a physician is required to handle prescriptions. The goal of these groups is supportive in the sense of helping the patient to master and cope with current problems. This does not mean that issues are ignored or handled with simple reassurance. A problem-solving approach with active use of homework tasks between sessions should be used.

One model that has been successfully used is to establish particular blocks of time each week, for example, an afternoon from 2:00 to 4:00 P.M., to which are assigned a substantial number of patients. The clinic is staffed by two outpatient staff members who are well connected with community resources. The patients may come at varying frequencies but always to their own afternoon clinic. Those recently discharged or threatening decompensation may come weekly, whereas others who have been stabilized on long-term medication may come monthly or even quarterly. For all of them, this is their home base. Over time, there is enough intermingling that they get to know most members of the extendable group population. Coffee and maybe cookies are provided, and serious talk about how things are going is expected. Such a program provides the structure for "transference to an institution." The afternoon clinic continues forever, even though the staff members may change as well as many of the patients. It remains as a supportive resource to be used as required. At the same time, it provides coverage for large numbers of patients with efficient use of staff time (78).

In this sort of clinic, there is a constant need for medication review and prescription renewal. A physician can attend for a portion of the clinic and take care of these requirements, if need be, seeing patients briefly privately. Sometimes medication needs are discussed as a portion of the group meeting. Where patients are being maintained on depot medication, they can leave the group to receive their injection in an adjacent medication office and then return. The advantage of this approach is that the group experience is at the heart of the clinic and the power of group cohesion is available to support patients dealing with a difficult illness. Family or friends can also be welcomed at these clinics, where they may learn useful methods of maximizing adaptation. Indeed, it provides a good forum for emphasizing the importance of maintaining a positive emotional tone in interactions with the patient, based on current understanding of the deleterious effects of a negative emotional environment.

Such a clinic provides a rich mixture of group therapeutic factors, primarily those drawn from the supportive cluster. Over time, these groups can deal with quite powerful personal issues, often having to do with coming to grips with diminished functioning and quasi-dependent status. For these types of groups, staff are best selected who have supportive and nurturing qualities, who prefer active solutions over psychological metaphors, and who know how to benignly but firmly set limits.

Self-help Groups

More people experience the effects of group participation through membership in self-help groups than in formal psychotherapy groups. Self-help groups span a wide variety of target populations usually defined on the basis of an illness or circumstance—for example, substance abuse, eating disorders, affective disorders, stroke patients, bereavement, family violence, or incest. Some of these programs focus on behavior management, others primarily provide an accepting and supportive environment. Because of the homogeneity provided by the selection criteria, these groups tend to be highly cohesive. Most are not led by professionals and are not leader centered (79).

There has been a belated recognition by the professional community that such groups offer important support for successful coping. This is primarily due to the "morale" cluster of therapeutic factors, although each organization has its own unique characteristics. Because of the homogeneity factor, self-help groups can be very effective in targeting dysfunctional behavior: "It takes one to know one," "I used to try that trick, but it won't work." On the other hand, these same processes may encourage collusion in the avoidance of central issues. Membership in the group can become the primary source of personal identification: "I am a . . . " This may be initially helpful, but eventually restricting. One basic, if unresolved, question has to do with the criteria for determining when formal therapy can be a useful adjunct or replacement to self-help activities.

It is best for the professional to avoid close involvement in the day-to-day activities of self-help organizations. They operate with well-established guidelines that do not need professional tampering. At the same time, a respectful attitude and a working relationship will encourage open communication, which can facilitate referrals in both directions.

Summary

This chapter pulls together a number of issues related to the implementation of group therapy in service delivery systems. The positive outcome literature together with characteristics of the pace of patient improvement suggest that time-limited groups can provide an important contribution that is both effective and efficient. The nature of groups may vary considerably, and it is essential that the type of group be matched to the needs of the program.

CHAPTER 15

Ethics and Supervision

This chapter considers the professional aspects of being a group therapist. General ethical guidelines promulgated by such professional bodies as the American Psychiatric Association or the American Psychological Association form the basis for clinical standards of practice. Implications of the group setting call for expansion of some of these ethical guidelines, particularly regarding confidentiality. Following this, some ideas about how to get the most out of supervision are presented. Training standards in group psychotherapy are briefly described.

Ethical Issues for the Group Therapist

The group psychotherapist, as opposed to a group facilitator or a group consultant, is functioning as a mental health care professional. This brings with it the social role obligations of the "healer." The fundamental expectations of this ancient role are that the professional will be knowledgeable, well intentioned, and responsible to act in the patient's best interest. The treatment environment is expected to be safe and supportive and, above all, should not make matters worse. The patient is entitled to be treated with dignity and respect and to have an opportunity of participating in decisions regarding care on a basis of reasonable knowledge (80).

These traditions do not mean that the therapist should or will like all patients nor agree with some of the things they do. It does carry with it the expectation that the professional will strive to behave toward each patient in a neutral and nonjudgmental fashion.

Confidentiality

A fundamental tenet of the psychotherapeutic condition is a belief that all information revealed will be held in confidentiality. This implies that only under carefully specified circumstances will information identifiable with a given patient be repeated outside of the therapeutic setting. There may be a greater tendency to talk about groups than about individual therapy. In one sense, the confidentiality barrier between doctor and patient has already been broken by the group situation, leading to a greater sense of laxity. There are a number of guidelines that can be used in addressing the question of confidentiality.

Talking with fellow professionals. Think carefully before talking about therapeutic matters even in a professional setting. When doing so, be extremely careful about expunging all identifiers and be sure that the material is being presented in a professional matter. With a group of colleagues, it may be easy to get into an escalating one-upmanship recitation of "war stories." Remember that everything you say reveals your respect for your patient's integrity and your attitudinal position as a professional. The life of a psychotherapist can be a lonely one, and opportunities to discuss clinical work and its stresses may be limited. Do not try to address that through stray conversation. If you need to discuss a case, even just to ventilate your frustration, use a peer who understands you and your situation, and talk with some degree of privacy.

Harmful attitudes. Attitudes conveying the impression that the therapist is manipulating, demeaning, or infantilizing the patient reflect a fundamental error in conceptualizing the doctor/patient relationship. Professionals have not been licensed to control or take advantage of others, but to assist them in mastering difficult situations. A critical or disparaging attitude, even in conversations with peers, suggests that therapeutic perspective has been lost. These sorts of attitudes are associated with poor outcome and a higher incidence of negative effects (81).

Public places. Avoid case discussions in public places. Elevators and cafeterias in medical centers are notorious for unfortunate leaks of confidentiality. There is no justification for discussion of clinical material in nonprofessional circles except for general theoretical statements or perhaps reference to one's successful treatment of 759 cases of serial murderers. Enticing tidbits should not be used to enliven conversation at cocktail parties. Some of the listeners may themselves be in, or have been in, therapy, and such comments can be damaging to the general reputation of the profession, to say nothing of your own reputation.

Clinical records.   The medical record may be subpoenaed. The purpose of this official record is to document and justify assessment and management decisions. It is not necessary to include a wealth of specific intimate details that would occasion embarrassment or more if they became public knowledge. In psychotherapeutic work, it is recurrent patterns that are important, not specific details. Some psychotherapists keep private process notes for short-term use and enter only significant management decisions or general progress reports in the official record.

Reports to others.   A similar principle can be applied to information sent to referral sources or follow-up services. This is particularly important when communicating with nonpsychiatric physicians or non–mental health agencies. Their ideas about the use of confidential information may be quite different from yours. It is best to write such letters mindful that they may be shown to the patient and may be read by clerical staff with minimal confidentiality guidelines.

Group member confidentiality.   The issue of confidentiality in groups is more complex. In Chapter 7, confidentiality was included as one important topic in pretherapy preparation. It is quite unusual for group confidentiality to be broken by members. As a preventive move, it is useful to reinforce the theme of confidentiality in early sessions or after a particularly significant piece of information has been revealed. The question of the legal status of information obtained by group members about each other is poorly tested in the courts.

Phone calls and emergencies.   If the therapist has contact with a group member between sessions, is it appropriate to share some or all of the information with the group? Sometimes phone contact is a benign matter of necessary arrangements, time conflicts, need for medication review, or so on. But phone calls often reflect a member's need to establish a special relationship with the therapist, to get extra recognition or favored status. As such, they must be classified as group issues involving the highly charged question of where one stands in the therapist's regard. The therapist must be alert to this dimension. Similarly, "emergencies" often happen at difficult times in the group and represent a tactic to defuse the issues or obtain extra therapist attention. In general, if the phone call or emergency relates to events in the group or topics under discussion there, then all efforts should be made to introduce it at the next session. Preferably, the patient can understand that this is indicated and do so spontaneously. The therapist must walk a fine line between breaking trust with the individual and ignoring the underlying importance of the event for the group. Careful clinical judgment must be applied. If outside contacts become a habit, then the ground rules need to be clearly specified and all such occurrences treated as extensions of the group session.

Taping. The use of audio- or videotaping in teaching or supervision is valuable; however, clear guidelines must be established regarding this practice. Group members have a right to know who has access to recordings. In general, access should be restricted to the involved clinician and a supervisor. It is wise to erase all tapes promptly after they have been reviewed unless they are being kept for a specific purpose. This avoids accidental exposure. One convenient method is to automatically erase and reuse tapes after a given time period from the recording date, perhaps after 2 or 3 weeks.

   Therapists are responsible for ensuring that all videotapes of their clinical work are regularly erased, particularly if they are leaving the clinical service. Routine storage of clinical tapes for unspecified use in the future should be discouraged. Such material is seldom utilized if it is not properly cataloged and is open to inappropriate use by persons unfamiliar with the clinical situation. When tapes are to be used for research or education purposes, special consent forms are required. This includes use of videotapes at grand rounds or similar educational settings where students or outside staff may not fully understand confidentiality issues. If recorded material is to be assembled into a permanent teaching package, it is wise to review it completely and expunge sensitive factual information (82).

Observation. Much group work is done in settings where sessions are routinely observed. Although observation rooms are a useful device for teaching and supervision, guidelines need to be established regarding access. This is best restricted to members of a small clinical team and supervisory personnel. The practice of "dropping in to see what's going on" should be prohibited. Professionals and students who do not work on the team should observe only with prior arrangements and clear guidelines. It is wise to discourage single observation visits. Such a practice fosters opportunities to take events out of context: "You should see some of things they do at Hospital X!" Often, therapeutic strategies are worked out over numerous sessions, and activity or inactivity may have meaning only in that larger time frame. A single observation experience may give quite distorted impressions about the clinical service and about learning group therapy.

Duty to warn or inform. Occasionally, information emerges in group sessions that must be reported elsewhere. This is a serious and delicate matter. Such information usually concerns potential danger to others, or information regarding family abuse patterns. Concerns about an increase in suicide risk must be followed up by the therapist if not in the group session itself, then immediately after. Sometimes information concerns social dangers such as impaired professionals or impaired drivers or pilots. The approach to these matters is no different than that in other therapy settings. The fact that such material arises in a group context does not alter the professional responsibility to act appropriately.

Sexual Involvement

Therapy groups tend to have a more egalitarian and open quality than individual office visits. This may stimulate patient fantasies regarding intimacy with the therapist or other group members. The therapist needs to be particularly alert to such themes. Care should be taken that familiarity or touching is not misinterpreted. As in all sensitive issues, such concerns should be carefully but firmly introduced into the discussion.

The therapist also may be susceptible to personal romantic responses regarding group members. Involvement with patients is properly coming under increasing scrutiny by professional organizations. The leader is in a position of sanctioned power and control. Personal involvement with patients is a violation of the responsibilities of that role. When fantasies of intimacy with patients occur, the therapist must immediately take this as a danger signal. If such attention does not dampen them, then a colleague or supervisor should be consulted for further discussions. It is inevitable that such ideas will from time to time occur. The professional has a responsibility to address them quickly and thoroughly.

Patient Autonomy

The issue of patient autonomy is fundamental to the question of the power balance in psychotherapy. Consider the following issues that occur almost daily in a clinical setting. Is the leader called John or Dr. Doe in the group? Would, or should, it make a difference? Who should set the goals for therapy? Is psychotherapy a process of education or a process of treatment, or both? Should psychotherapy be designed to help the individual rebel against and change his or her environment? Or should it be more concerned with adaptation and learning to accept difficult circumstances? Is the patient able to manage independently, or will excessively optimistic therapist expectations lead to an experience of failure? What is the therapist's influence on the patient in terms of social responsibility? Is guilt a good sign or an indication of unresolved conflict? What is the best balance between a sense of responsibility for others and taking care of self? Does the therapist view people as basically good and with strengths in need of development, or as people basically conflicted or sinful and in need of correction? You may want to add to this list of questions.

Although there are no absolute answers to these issues, therapeutic styles are influenced by the approach to questions of belief or faith. Every therapist has a position regarding religion, sexuality, abortion, marriage, and personal responsibility. What role do such items of belief play in your therapy? How do you react to patient decisions that seem unwise, disastrous, or morally wrong? How much "leakage" of your opinions occurs without your being aware of it? In one way or another, the answers to these questions effect the control the therapist will have over the direction of patient change (83).

The history of psychiatric treatment is a somewhat sad litany of efforts by well-meaning practitioners to treat the major mental illnesses with inadequate methods. Often, these involved coercive techniques prescribed authoritatively. Enthusiasm often exceeded demonstrated effectiveness. Such phenomena are not lacking today in regard to both biologic and psychotherapeutic approaches. It is easy for the student or practitioner to adopt the views of prominent authorities and apply them without careful clinical judgment. If done so with enthusiasm, the patient may be exposed to considerable pressure to see the solution to a problem in terms of the theories of the therapist. The professional needs to be very careful that the results are indeed in the patient's best interests. From the other side, the question is whether to have faith that patients will change in ways that are best for them.

These questions of patient autonomy apply to all types of psychotherapy. They seem particularly relevant to the group therapy context because motivation and pressure for change is amplified by group peer pressure. These forces may be even more insidious than influence exerted in individual therapy. Not only can the combined opinion expressed by six or eight members be very convincing, but it may be interpreted as carrying implications for acceptance by the group. You will recall that a cohesive group is defined as having the ability to influence its members.

The nature of group influence may reflect transitory group phenomena that can distort perspective. For example, a group approaching issues of intimacy may displace some of these concerns onto outside circumstances and encourage a member to become involved with some outside person about whom the group has only fragmentary knowledge, with potentially unfortunate results. The rules of society or the workplace are not necessarily the rules of the group. The therapist needs to monitor the degree to which specific suggestions are being used in the group. In general, advice giving is characteristic of early groups and gives way with time to a more flexible style in which issues are examined for meaning and clarification more than specific solutions.

The guidelines in this book concerning careful assessment and clarification of goals, as well as pretherapy preparation regarding how the group will operate, all serve to forewarn the patient. As the group progresses, the therapist is in a position to monitor for inappropriate effects of group pressure and to specifically address the issue if there appears to be danger of poorly thought-out decisions. The task is not to deny the right of personal choice but rather to caution about major decisions in the midst of the therapeutic process (84).

It is appropriate for the therapist to raise questions in the group regarding the effect of group pressure. Some strategy to encourage a delay in acting on group suggestions may be useful. In the final analysis, overt or covert influence is rampant in groups, originating both from the leader and from the members. This is generally benign and can stimulate a personal reassessment process in members. One advantage of the stage ideas in Chapter 4 is that a group that has mastered the tasks of stages 1 and 2 should have the ability to support and agree, as well as competence to challenge and assert. Nonetheless, it behooves therapists to regularly ask themselves where they really stand on the question of patient autonomy.

Capitalizing on Supervision

Didactic theory and experiential learning are useful for a beginning group therapist, but systematic supervision is the single most important ingredient in developing psychotherapeutic skills. Many experienced group psychotherapists also seek out supervision opportunities of a formal or informal nature to keep them alert to skills maintenance (85).

A specific supervisor should be identified. It is not sufficient for a new group therapist to sample opinions from various staff or peers and then pick and choose from their off-the-cuff suggestions. This process may only serve to reinforce naive interpretations because ideas may be rejected that do not coincide with those of the therapist. Facts may be presented in a selective fashion that guarantees a self-fulfilling response. This process may go on quite outside of the full awareness of the trainee. Not surprisingly, areas of skill development that are most difficult are often those that are easiest to avoid.

Trainees should negotiate, even demand, a consistent supervisory resource if one is not provided. It is preferable that the name of the supervisor be clearly identified on the patient's records as the Attending of Record and that patients are informed that their therapist has a supervisor with whom all clinical information will be shared. This forestalls later revelations of these facts, which might prove embarrassing. It also ensures that the supervisor takes the job seriously. The critical issue is that a mechanism be in place for ensuring consistent and responsible supervisory input.

For more experienced therapists, various other methods of supervision may be organized. In a large service delivery system, team meetings may provide a mechanism for review of groups. Some professionals organize small groups of colleagues who meet regularly to discuss therapeutic management problems, with or without a designated leader. At the very least, it is useful to identify another colleague with whom you explicitly agree to discuss problematic cases. Time for informal discussion about the work and its stresses serves an important maintenance function. Constant psychotherapeutic involvement can be isolating, and biases or tensions may build gradually without the individual being quite aware of why the work has become less satisfying. Sometimes these reparative functions are accomplished, at least in part, at professional meetings where opportunities for workshop or small group discussions are available.

A distinction must be made between intensive training supervision and general caseload management. In the former situation, it is preferable that the supervisor be outside regular administrative channels so that the therapist can feel comfortable in acknowledging questions, deficits, and uncertainties without such material becoming part of a formal training or service file entry. A certain amount of "regression in the service of learning" is an inevitable part of developing clinical skills, and some safe outlet for this is important.

Serious lapses in memory and reporting can occur through the sole use of process notes or session summaries. Group psychotherapy involves interpersonal skills, not just intellectual understanding. The use of live material whether it be through observation, videotape, or audiotape draws attention back to basics. Unfortunately, supervision may focus on higher-order inferential interpretative matters without adequate regard for the reliability of the facts on which they are based. The opportunity of replaying group events with time to stop and consider them is an enormous advantage in developing sensitivity to process events. Simply watching a playback provides the therapist with an automatic corrective process. Going over tapes with a peer is relatively nonthreatening and very helpful. Reviewing them with a supervisor may be initially anxiety provoking but has important payoff. Inexpensive home video equipment can operate at room light levels with adequate sound pickup. It is also helpful for teachers and supervisors to allow students to see them at work.

Group psychotherapy, like family therapy, exposes the therapist to the power of "system suction." This refers to the pull of social systems on participants to understand events in terms of the group's solution to its problems. For example, a group may be experiencing difficulty in coming to grips with conflict or the expression of critical or angry responses between members. The group solution to this stress may be to displace negative affect onto an external focus such as university authorities (in student health centers), the nursing system (in inpatient groups), or cold and distant fathers (in eating disorders groups). It may be quite difficult for the therapist to avoid being drawn into these rationales, because they generally contain a grain of truth. The extent to which the material is being used as resistance may be missed. An opportunity to review the session verbally or via videotape may be sufficient to regain a systems perspective.

One major function of the supervision process is to provide a neutral field for exploration of group-level phenomena. A systematic review of major session themes allows an opportunity for a dispassionate second opinion and subsequent identification of subtle mechanisms. In Chapter 16, a system for recording group sessions is outlined. It will help the therapist to identify thematic developments and the relative contributions of different members to these themes. The process of thinking through and writing down major themes and discussing them with a supervisor is a major step toward resisting group suction.

There are some advantages to having group supervision in a small group. The process of the supervision group itself constitutes a useful alerting mechanism. At times, the process in the supervision group may come to resemble features of the groups being supervised, giving added impetus to the discussion. Having supervision with one's peers also makes it easier to discuss the uncertainties and ambiguities that are an inevitable part of learning to do group therapy. The leadership style in a supervisory group may form a model of therapist behavior that can be usefully applied in the clinical groups. A small-group supervision format allows learning from the experiences of several groups and thus expands the experiential base. It also is efficient use of supervisor time.

One problem with group supervision is the difficulty in maintaining some degree of familiarity with events in each of the groups being supervised. Group therapy entails the application of therapeutic skills in a complex field. Therefore, attention to the specifics must constitute an important part of supervision for the beginning group therapist. Trying to cover more than two or three groups makes this difficult. For the more advanced therapist, supervision may be conducted in larger groups where there is no effort to deal in a systematic manner with the specific events of the groups. Rather, the supervision group itself is seen as an indirect analog to the therapy groups, and the supervision is more akin to experiential training than to detailed process examination.

The development of group therapeutic skills may be considered under three broad categories: perceptual, conceptual, and executive.

Perceptual skills.   Is the therapist able to recognize phenomena that are happening in a group? Sitting in the leader's chair is inevitably accompanied by some anxiety, and the new therapist may become temporarily unskilled in making observations. The group may be seen only as a single entity and the contributions of individuals missed. Or the therapist may focus on individual members and miss general group effects. The use of observation or video playback is very helpful in developing perceptual skills. It is recommended that residents learning group psychotherapy keep videotapes of the first two or three sessions of the group. Reviewing them several months later is an educational exercise in detecting early leakage of important themes that appear overtly only much later in the course of therapy.

Conceptual analysis.   The second category of skills has to do with giving meaning to the information that is perceived. The beginning therapist usually gravitates toward explanations that deal with individual motivations or psychopathology. It is important to develop an understanding of the theory of group-level phenomena to counterbalance this. The essential question is How can one understand why these people are doing these things together at this time? In group therapy, as in individual therapy, the actual process of interacting in the therapy setting probably constitutes the most important change-inducing experience. By focusing on trying to understand the here-and-now process going on between the members within the group, the therapist has access to material that is of direct relevance to therapeutic outcome. Writing up the session and discussing it with a supervisor facilitates the acquisition of a group perspective.

Executive action.   The third major skill area is that of executive action. Having perceived and conceptualized the group events, what is the best therapeutic response? This is usually the least controversial of the three because working through the conceptual issues often leads to inevitable conclusions regarding what is required. This may involve subtleties of clinical judgment regarding timing or emphasis. Sometimes it simply involves doing what must be done.

Skill Development and Supervision

These three levels of skill development are useful to consider in the context of supervision. They form a hierarchy of expertise. That is why it is important that beginning group therapists be observed. Later, with more experience, perceptions can be relied on and the focus can shift to discussing the meaning of group events and possible approaches. There is an understandable pressure for beginning therapists to move immediately to the question of what to do now. Fast advice is seldom useful. The levels of perception and conceptualization must be reviewed, at which point the action implications may reveal themselves. Looking at videotapes of sessions or going through a detailed debriefing with cotherapists, observers, or your own process notes will help.

Having done this, the trainee is in a better position to take to a supervisor a properly formulated question. This may be couched early on in terms of, "So much was happening, I couldn't make much sense of it." A detailed recall of the events will help to focus on perceptual skills. A later question might be "I saw such and such going on, but I wasn't sure how to understand it." Here, a discussion of theoretical issues would be appropriate. Is the behavior best seen as an example of a recurrent pattern based on individual psychological pathology? Is it best understood as a function of the individual member's relationship to you the therapist? Might it be seen as part of a larger group process in which the individual is playing a particular role fostered by the group members? Or could it be the resultant of several of these factors coming together at one point in time? A third level might be introduced with the question, "I am pretty sure I understood what was happening, but I found myself frozen and unsure exactly how to respond." In this case, exploration of the sources of anxiety might be helpful. Various executive options might be considered and tried out in the supervision room.

You as a trainee can help your supervisor by thinking through what level needs to be addressed. Supervisors may consider a trainee a skilled individual therapist and not recognize that he or she needs to begin with the basics in regard to groups. It is probably more fun for supervisors to speculate at the conceptual level and assume that the facts are accurate. For your own development, you may need to remind them where you stand. It is understandable that a new group therapist will want all the answers at once. An important part of the learning process is to think though the issues without expecting absolute answers.

The supervisory experience, whether it be individual or group in nature, is also a developing relationship. It needs to move through the same developmental stages as therapy groups and often does so in parallel. It can be a useful part of learning to go through this experience yourself and to assist in its development within the supervisory setting. This is based on a willingness to talk openly and honestly about your experiences as a therapist in your own group and about the process in the supervision setting, about both your ideas and your emotional reactions. These are the same instructions given to patients embarking on a course of psychotherapy. The recommendations may prove equally as difficult to consistently implement. The supervisee has just as much responsibility to work on these issues as the supervisor.

Supervision provides an opportunity to learn more about the professional role. The process of therapy and the process of supervision have different goals but similar processes. Think of using your supervision sessions not just for information or specific suggestions but for understanding attitudes about patient care and the balance between support and confrontation. Supervision sessions also provide experience in tolerating a degree of ambiguity regarding exactly what to do, the same dilemma your patients may be experiencing.

Doing your homework before taking therapeutic issues to your supervisor has advantages. In supervision as in psychotherapy, it is a positive sign associated with good outcome when homework is done and reported. The group report form in Chapter 16 is designed with that in mind. By forcing yourself to describe each item succinctly, you will be in a position to identify issues that need to be addressed. At the same time, such organization will be highly motivating to your supervisor, who sees you constructively making use of the supervision opportunity.

Above all, if supervision is not going satisfactorily, that fact needs to be addressed. Often, it is related to a misalignment in terms of expectations, which may be readily addressed. Sometimes it reflects a difference in theoretical orientation. For example, a trainee whose experience has been primarily with the metaphors of cognitive behavioral therapy may be matched with a supervisor who utilizes the metaphors of psychoanalysis. Each may see the other as avoiding important dimensions, without recognizing the common core to both theoretical positions. Perhaps most commonly, problems between supervisor and supervisee reflect difficulties in the therapy group being supervised. Looking at these supervision issues may suddenly illuminate what is going wrong in the therapy. In short, address the supervision process just as you would address the psychotherapy process, including notes.

Training of the Group Therapist

Basic standards for group psychotherapy training have been developed by the American Group Psychotherapy Association (AGPA). The components of a training program may be described under four headings: didactic material, observation of groups, personal group experience, and supervised practice (86).

Didactic material.   This book contains an introductory level of information going somewhat beyond the AGPA core curriculum. The references provide a reasonable sampling of major authors and theoretical positions. The AGPA requires a 12-hour core curriculum of a standard nature, followed by further courses for a total of 90 didactic hours. Regular reading of the *International Journal of Group Psychotherapy*, and *Group*, the journal of the Eastern Group Psychotherapy Society, will keep the practitioner abreast of current ideas.

Observation.   An active group environment produces a large amount of clinical information. Observing a group provides an opportunity to practice integrating this material. This should be done over a number of sessions in order to see the same members interacting around different issues and to see the evolution of the group work over time. Observation also helps to desensitize the beginning therapist to tolerating an intensive group atmosphere. This is particularly the case where the observer sits in the group room. The AGPA does not specify this training experience, but it is a standard component of most educational programs.

Personal experience in groups.   Personal experience as a member of a group is an important component of training. There is a spectrum of opinion regarding experiential learning versus psychotherapy. Some training programs expect their students to be fully participating members of a therapy group. Most training programs recommend participation in an experiential training group in which personal issues from outside the group are discouraged and the main focus is on the here-and-now group process. The AGPA criteria call for 60 hours of group participation, some of which can be obtained in the context of conferences or workshops (87).

Supervision.   As reviewed earlier in this chapter, supervision should be systematic, regular, and extended over time. It should deal not just with clinical emergencies, but with the day-to-day mechanics of running groups. Supervisors should themselves be experienced in group psychotherapy so that both individual dynamics and group-level phenomena can be addressed. The AGPA stipulates a minimum of 60 hours leading one or more patient groups and 25 hours supervising this experience.

Training in Individual Therapy

Because group psychotherapy requires the application of the principles of individual therapy, training in individual work should be expected as part of the preparation of the group therapist. Group work requires an additional layer of theory and technique above and beyond that needed for individual therapy. The group psychotherapist must be able to integrate these two perspectives. The family therapist generally finds the transition to group work theoretically easy although frustrating in application because of the need to develop a new social system rather than using an established one.

Summary

The group therapist is subject to the usual expectations of professional ethics. The open nature of groups calls for particular care in regard to issues of confidentiality. For the beginning therapist, the availability of supervision is most important. The use of observation or videotape techniques enhances learning. The process of supervision is bilateral, and the trainee can do much to maximize its effectiveness. National training guidelines in group psychotherapy are available.

CHAPTER **16**

Records and Measures

This chapter provides a method for keeping group records that should be of value to the clinician as well as the medical records department. It also introduces several clinical methods for measuring change and for monitoring group process, including simple forms for group members to complete as well as forms for use by therapists or observers.

Group Records

Good record keeping is a necessary part of clinical practice. The recording of group therapy events is a more complex task than recording individual sessions. The group report form discussed in the next section should be completed immediately after the session while the experience and the sense of involvement are still alive. A delay of even an hour produces a drop in the accuracy and immediacy of the records. Trying to write up a group session the next day or a week later is not only unsatisfactory in terms of recording events accurately, but is also less satisfying in terms of reviewing for yourself the important aspects of the session. Time should be set aside to write up the session. Fifteen minutes is a bare minimum, and for a new therapist, 30 minutes is more realistic. This time should not be squashed in while keeping the next patient waiting. It should be considered as part of the time allotment for the group and carefully preserved as such.

A postgroup discussion involving cotherapists or observers immediately after the session is invaluable. It provides an opportunity to integrate the group events, to identify connections not seen at the time, and to recognize major themes. It is a good time to focus systematically on group-level ideas and the participation of each member. It is also an opportunity to react personally to the group events and, by understanding them, put them in perspective.

Just as time is needed at the end of a group session, so a few minutes should to be taken before each session to review notes from the preceding group. The group report form is designed with that function in mind. The purpose of spending a few minutes recalling the previous session is to place yourself back into the group atmosphere. This is often a problem. Patients may spend hours mulling over what happened in the preceding session and come in ready to continue where they left off. Therapists, on the other hand, have seen a week of patients in between. Many of these are likely to have generally similar themes and require related therapeutic strategies. Everyone has had the experience of catching oneself halfway through an intervention with the sickening realization that, although the intent may have been correct, the facts belonged to another patient. A few minutes spent before the start of a group session reorienting oneself to the "lay of the land" at the end of the last session is very helpful.

Group Report Form

The challenge for the group therapist in maintaining records is to capture issues pertinent to each individual member as well as to the entire group. At the same time, records need to be brief enough that they do not take an inordinately long time to record. Brevity also facilitates a fast review before the next session.

The one-page group report form in the Appendix is a satisfactory compromise. Basic identifying information is entered at the top: the group, date, and session number, as well as the names of the therapist(s) and any observers. The names of members and therapist(s) are placed in the circle of boxes in accordance with the seating arrangement during the group. Within each box, summarize the main issues raised by the individual, including the therapist. By allowing only limited space, the clinician must summarize important themes and not get into too much detail. This can be a salutary experience in condensation that drives compulsive therapists wild. Before leaving the top part of the form, draw lines between the boxes indicating the strength of interaction between each member of the group, including the therapist. Triple lines indicate a heavy connection, double lines some significant interaction, single lines only weak communication, and no lines negligible contact between the individuals. This simple directional pattern is quite revealing of group process patterns. The remainder of the page is used for group-level comments.

1. *Major themes.*   Stand back from the group and consider the few principal thematic topics that were discussed during the session. Understandably, this will eliminate a lot of detail and focus only on the main issues around which the session was organized. In most sessions, this will amount to three or four areas. It is useful to provide brief examples and to try to identify triggering events that resulted in a shift of theme.

2. *Critical incidents.*   This section enlarges on the idea of themes. List and briefly describe the few episodes that stand out as being of particular importance. These are usually heralded by the emergence of strong affect. Go around the group and think of events that seemed relevant to each member. Critical incidents often involve self-disclosure, insightful breakthroughs, an important exchange between two members, or a unified group reaction such as an attack on one member or the leader. These episodes can be briefly identified as an aide-mémoire for later use.

3. *Therapist issues.*   Identify major events involving the therapist, including evidence for transferential and countertransferential reactions. A brief comment might be made about the main features of therapist intervention style. If there are cotherapists, review the quality of their collaboration.

4. *Supervision comments.*   Include here ideas from the postgroup discussion or formal supervision session. These might involve ideas about the meaning of some group events, or thoughts on technique or therapeutic strategy.

5. *For next session.*   After having thought through the session in order to write it up, and after having discussed it with observers or a supervisor, make a list of issues to consider before entering the next session. These may relate to structural issues such as attendance or tardiness, content areas for follow-up, issues that predictably may come up or should be brought up, aspects of technique to consider, strategies concerning any given patient such as the need

for more support or more confrontation, aspects of the group climate or norms to be addressed, and so on. Sometimes these are hot ideas generated immediately after the session that should not be lost. The list should not be too long, probably five or six items is enough.

The group report form has been intentionally kept to one page in order to force the therapist to abstract themes. The result is more efficient and effective group records rather than lengthy anecdotal summaries that may occupy several pages but are lacking in focus.

Use of Structured Measures in Clinical Work

The psychotherapeutic aspect of psychiatric care has been criticized for its heavy reliance on clinical judgment. There are increasing pressures to justify the cost-effectiveness of services. Sophisticated consumers are now more comfortable asking for information regarding effectiveness. Fortunately, psychotherapy research is entering a phase of consolidation in which there is general agreement about major dimensions to be studied. Appropriate instruments are becoming available (88).

Formal measurement techniques involve the patient in the treatment process and encourage open feedback about the course of treatment. They help to introduce an objective perspective and may give the patient some indication about the complexity of the change process. Well-selected instruments help to establish connections between the therapy procedures and outcome.

To use these measures, the therapist needs to become familiar with the instruments, their format and theoretical origins, and what sort of results can be expected. With this background, the procedures can be presented to the patient with confidence. A hesitant or mildly deprecating attitude will discourage compliance and affect reliability of the results. Patients should be told clearly what is involved and how much time this will require. Their participation as collaborators in understanding themselves and the treatment should be enlisted. They need to be assured that the results will be handled responsibly, and, where possible, they should have the opportunity to discuss results with the clinician. The measures described in this chapter have been selected for their simplicity and relevance to the therapeutic task. With a careful approach, the great majority of patients are not only willing to help in data collection, they enjoy the process (89).

Measuring Change in Patients

The process of change in psychotherapy is complex and involves a number of dimensions and viewpoints from the highly subjective to the austerely objective. Because the goal of group therapy is to promote change in the individual, methods to measure change are similar to those used for individual therapy. Such a battery should include some measures that are focused on interpersonal functioning because this is central to the group approach (90).

When setting up a change measures battery, the following criteria need to be considered: 1) multiple measures representing different aspects of functioning, 2) a combination of subjective impressions and objective behavioral measures, 3) individualized measures along with standardized instruments, and 4) several sources of assessment information.

These criteria may be organized into the matrix shown in Table 16-1. Though this table may appear complex at first glance, the information is really part of the usual clinical assessment data base. The use of structured methods to collect some types of data does not replace the usual clinical history, nor is it intended to replace clinical judgment. Structured assessment can be usefully used for screening purposes and as a double check on clinical impressions. Most patients report that these procedures are easy to complete, make clinical sense, and sometimes pick up issues that they had not thought of stating directly. The battery described here would take the average patient less than an hour to complete and would involve only a few minutes of clinician time. The instruments can be given as a handout to take home or can be completed in the office. The latter is preferable though not essential. Completion at home sometimes turns into a family project, which makes the results interesting but possibly inaccurate for the individual. Most of the measures can also be effectively administered on a microcomputer. Several studies indicate that patients enjoy this process and report that it is easier to answer truthfully to a dispassionate machine that in the context of a clinical interview.

Demographic data sheet.   Demographic variables are standard items on most intake forms. Such information not only allows you to report clinical work systematically, it also may provide some guidelines in determining the type of treatment and likelihood of response. Basic demographic data include age, sex, marital status, educational level, and occupational category. The last two items can be used to calculate social class (91).

Table 16-1. Components of change measures battery

Type of information	Source of information		
	Patient	Therapist	Clinical record
Demographics/ statistics			Data sheet Service utilization
Symptoms	SCL-90	SCL-Analogue	
Social functioning	Social Adjustment Scale		
Target goals	Target goals	Target goals	
Global functioning		Global Assessment Scale	

Note. SCL-90 = Symptom Checklist 90.

Service utilization statistics. One objective method for measuring successful outcome is a comparison, before and after, of the use of treatment resources. Adding up the number of office visits, the number of hospital admissions, the number of days in the hospital, or the number of emergency room visits in the 6- or 12-month period immediately preceding and immediately following treatment termination gives a "hard" measure of treatment effect. Such information is easily obtained from hospital and outpatient clinic record systems or can be extracted from the records of a private office. Studies indicate a substantial drop in general medical as well as psychiatric visits after psychiatric treatment termination (92).

Symptom Checklist 90 (SCL-90-R). This 90-item self-report symptom inventory is the latest version of the Cornell Medical Index. There is a high degree of correlation between the SCL-90-R subscale scores and comparable Minnesota Multiphasic Personality Inventory (MMPI) dimensions. Results are expressed in nine symptom dimensions: somatization, obsessive-compulsive, interpersonal sensitivity, depression, anxiety, hostility, phobic anxiety, paranoid ideation, and psychoticism. A Global Severity Index gives an overall measure of symptom status. The SCL is also available in a shorter 53-item version that yields a satisfactory Global Severity Index (93).

Social Adjustment Scale (SAS). This 60-item self-report instrument assesses the patient's functioning in a number of social roles.

The SAS was developed for use with a depressed outpatient population. It has the major advantage of being available in a self-report format. Subscores are obtained in the areas of work, social and pleasure activities, and relationship with extended family, as well as the roles of spouse, parent, and member of a family unit. Items tap four categories of adjustment: performance at expected tasks, finer aspects of interpersonal relations, friction with others, and internal feelings and satisfactions. An overall total score is also calculated (94).

Target goals. The identification of target goals offers an opportunity for patient and therapist, together or separately, to establish some directions for treatment. This idea of a problem-oriented approach is particularly important for brief therapy, in which a greater degree of focus is required. It is also an excellent method for priming the patient to think in terms of personal change. A simple format is presented in the Appendix. Goals can be assessed at intervals. Often, as therapy progresses, the nature of treatment goals shifts, and new goals can be added to the list as required.

Global Assessment of Functioning Scale. This scale consists of a 90-point continuum with descriptive criteria at 10-point intervals (Table 16-2). It has recently been incorporated into Axis V of the multiaxial DSM-III-R system. The clinician simply selects the point on the scale at which the patient is currently functioning. This choice is based on a combination of three dimensions of psychopathology: impairment of everyday functioning in social relations, work, and leisure time; symptoms and reality testing; and potential for suicide or violence. It is a straightforward method for the clinician to make a global statement concerning assessment of the patient (95).

Interpersonal functioning. When considering change over time, it is useful to keep symptoms experienced by the patient quite separate from interpersonal behavior. It is not unusual for symptoms to improve but behavior to remain unchanged, perhaps related to environmental contingencies. Sometimes behavior improves dramatically, but complaints of symptoms persist. The measurement of personality and interpersonal behavior is a controversial area, one in which there is a diversity of strongly held opinions. The most widely used general instrument continues to be the MMPI, a lengthy 566-item questionnaire that includes scales related to both symptoms and behavior. A new version of the MMPI is scheduled for release in 1989.

Table 16-2. Global Assessment of Functioning Scale (GAF Scale)

Consider psychological, social, and occupational functioning on a hypothetical continuum of mental health-illness. Do not include impairment in functioning due to physical (or environmental) limitations. See p. 20 [of DSM-III-R] for instructions on how to use this scale.

Note: Use intermediate codes when appropriate, e.g., 45, 68, 72.

Code

90
|
|
|
81
Absent or minimal symptoms (e.g., mild anxiety before an exam), **good functioning in all areas, interested and involved in a wide range of activities, socially effective, generally satisfied with life, no more than everyday problems or concerns** (e.g., an occasional argument with family members).

80
|
|
71
If symptoms are present, they are transient and expectable reactions to psychosocial stressors (e.g., difficulty concentrating after family argument); **no more than slight impairment in social, occupational, or school functioning** (e.g., temporarily falling behind in school work).

70
|
|
61
Some mild symptoms (e.g., depressed mood and mild insomnia) **OR some difficulty in social, occupational, or school functioning** (e.g., occasional truancy, or theft within the household), **but generally functioning pretty well, has some meaningful interpersonal relationships.**

60
|
51
Moderate symptoms (e.g., flat affect and circumstantial speech, occasional panic attacks) **OR moderate difficulty in social, occupational, or school functioning** (e.g., few friends, conflicts with co-workers).

50
|
41
Serious symptoms (e.g., suicidal ideation, severe obsessional rituals, frequent shoplifting) **OR any serious impairment in social, occupational, or school functioning** (e.g., no friends, unable to keep a job).

40
|
|
|
|
31
Some impairment in reality testing or communication (e.g., speech is at times illogical, obscure, or irrelevant) **OR major impairment in several areas, such as work or school, family relations, judgment, thinking, or mood** (e.g., depressed man avoids friends, neglects family, and is unable to work; child frequently beats up younger children, is defiant at home, and is failing at school).

30
|
|
21
Behavior is considerably influenced by delusions or hallucinations OR serious impairment in communication or judgment (e.g., sometimes incoherent, acts grossly inappropriately, suicidal preoccupation) **OR inability to function in almost all areas** (e.g., stays in bed all day; no job, home, or friends).

20
|
|
11
Some danger of hurting self or others (e.g., suicide attempts without clear expectation of death, frequently violent, manic excitement) **OR occasionally fails to maintain minimal personal hygiene** (e.g., smears feces) **OR gross impairment in communication** (e.g., largely incoherent or mute).

10
|
1
Persistent danger of severely hurting self or others (e.g., recurrent violence) **OR persistent inability to maintain minimal personal hygiene OR serious suicidal act with clear expectation of death.**

0
Inadequate information.

Benjamin's Structural Analysis of Social Behavior (SASB) (96) has been used throughout the book as a general organizing structure for interpersonal behavior. SASB is also available for use as a patient questionnaire. A brief version can be completed regarding the patient's perception of important people in present and past circumstances. This gives a complex bidirectional picture: How I act and react with you and how you act and react with me.

Group Process Measures

In contrast to the many ways available to measure patient change, the number of satisfactory group process measures is quite limited. Most have been designed for formal research studies and require typed transcripts or highly trained raters. However, there are several measures that are thought provoking and helpful for augmenting clinical impressions about group process. These focus on specific dimensions that help to organize the development of clinical judgment (97).

As with change measures, it is useful to consider methods that have different perspectives on the group process. Instruments can also be used by staff observers or trainees in addition to group members and therapists as a technique to develop skill at looking objectively at group events. It is useful to consider measures that look at the group as a whole, such as group climate measures, as well as those that deal with specific parts of the group interaction, such as critical incidents or leader behavior. As with change measures, the few simple parameters in Table 16-3 may be used to organize the approach to measuring process events.

Table 16-3. Components of process measures battery

Type of information	Source of information		
	Patient	Therapist	Observer
Group climate	GCQ/GES	GCQ/GES	GCQ/GES
Group interaction		HIM-G	HIM-G
Critical incidents	Critical incident form		
Therapist behavior	GES	HIM-G	HIM-G

Note. GCQ = Group Climate Questionnaire.   GES = Group Environment Scale.   HIM = Hill Interaction Matrix.

The following instruments have all been used in clinical settings and are acceptable, indeed interesting, to patients and clinicians alike. They are concerned with aspects of group process that are directly linked to change-inducing mechanisms and therefore to outcome.

Group Climate Questionnaire (GCQ).   This is a brief 12-item questionnaire for completion at the end of a group session by patients, therapists, or observers (see Appendix). It may be used routinely as a postsession measure and can be conveniently coupled with a critical incident form. Three subscales are built into the GCQ:

1. *Engaged*: a positive working environment
2. *Conflict*: a negative atmosphere with anger and distrust
3. *Avoiding* of personal responsibility for group work

The results may be expressed as raw scores based on the mean of the items involved in a particular subscale, or they may be converted into standard scores that make greater allowance for the usual range obtained on each subscale (98).

Group Environment Scale (GES).   This instrument grew out of extensive work on the measurement of social environments. It is psychometrically well developed and contains 90 true/false statements. Ten subscale scores are calculated based on three categories of information: relationship dimensions (cohesion, leader support, expressiveness), personal growth dimensions (independence, task orientation, self-discovery, anger and aggression), and system maintenance dimensions (order and organization, leader control, innovation). This instrument is suitable for intermittent use in clinical groups but is somewhat long for regular use. One could use selective subscales more frequently, for example, the 9-item cohesion subscale has items dealing with the idea of attraction to and faith in the group. In addition, the leader support and leader control subscales reflect two important dimensions of leader behavior (99).

Both the GCQ and the GES represent attempts to capture the group atmosphere as something above and beyond the activities of any one person. This calls for tricky judgment decisions when, for example, the action is dominated by one person, or if two conflicting dimensions are both in evidence. For that reason, the scales are unidimensional, and it is not logically inconsistent to describe a group as being very engaged even though there may be quite a bit of conflict.

Figure 16-1 demonstrates what an "ideal" group might look like in terms of group development ideas. Stage 1 is characterized by a rising level of "engaged" and falling levels of "avoiding" with minimal "conflict." Stage 2 is heralded by awareness of avoiding followed by a breakthrough of conflict and lowered engaged. Once this has been mastered, the group experiences stronger engaged yet can tolerate conflict.

One aspect of member reports is of particular interest. Members will "see" the group according to different criteria. These may reflect personality style or that person's immediate experiences in the group. For whatever reason, this spread of responses among group members can be substantial. Some members may be identified who are viewing the group in increasingly negative terms. Some may seem out of step with the rest of the group. Such information may be useful to the therapist, not for definitive action, but to maintain a search for the meaning of such discrepancies. As a general principle, it is wise not to report individual group climate scores back to the group, but the information from the questionnaire can be used as a guide to the therapist seeking clarification.

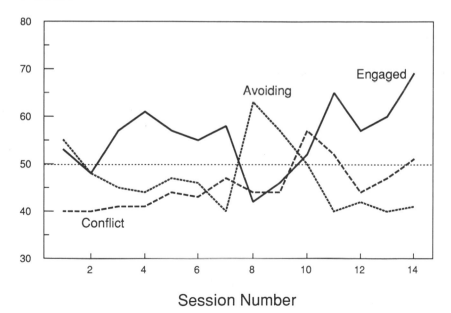

Figure 16-1. Group climate scores over first 14 sessions of a weekly outpatient group.

Critical incident reports.   In Chapter 10, the idea of critical incidents was used as a way of focusing on important group events. A critical incident form is a simple way of collecting similar impressions from group members. A sample is included in the Appendix along with the Group Climate Questionnaire. These free-form descriptions of important events as seen through the eyes of the members may help the therapist to understand the patients' perspectives. It may also alert the therapist to emerging dynamic theme issues. It is not unusual for members to "leak" issues on a critical incident form that rise to the verbal surface in the next session or two. It is helpful to think of critical incidents as representing the enactment of therapeutic factors, thus connecting them to a broader theoretical understanding. For practical purposes, it is adequate to use the broader clusters discussed in Chapter 3: supportive, self-revelation, learning from others, and psychological work factors (100).

Hill Interaction Matrix (HIM).   The HIM is a system for rating group events using four content and four process categories, as indicated in Figure 16-2. It is based on a theory of group effectiveness that assumes best results are achieved when personal issues are discussed in a confrontational manner by all group members. Accordingly, effective group work stems from interactions typical of the lower-right quadrant. A 72-item rating scale, the HIM-G, may be scored by the therapist or observer after a session. This is an excellent way to train residents or staff members to look critically at group interaction. It can also be used to categorize types of groups in a descriptive fashion. Within the HIM-G, 32 items relate specifically to therapist activities. These may be used to develop a description of leader style that can help beginning group leaders to conceptualize their activities (101).

SASB.   The theoretical ideas built into SASB are very suitable for analyzing group process. They may be used to categorize the group climate, critical incidents, specific interactions, or the activities of a given member or leader. In a recent transcript analysis of a group session, for example, it emerged that what looked like a productive working segment was in fact a battle royal over control issues.

Summary

This chapter has been based on ideas drawn from the research literature, material not commonly included in group therapy courses. As

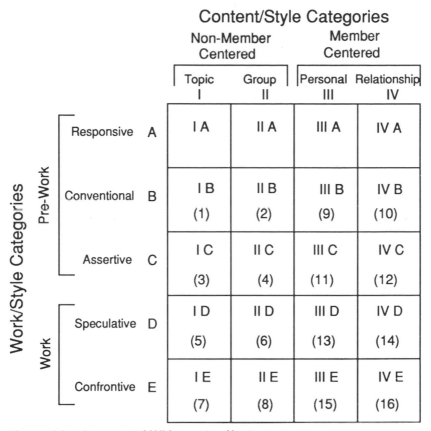

Figure 16-2. Categories of Hill Interaction Matrix.

Parloff noted, "The twin fields of psychotherapy and psychotherapy research have emerged, developed, and flourished in essentially untrammeled independence of each other" (102). There is increasing recognition that clinicians can be comfortable with the tools of clinical investigation, provided they do not interfere unduly with the therapeutic process. The intent is not to make clinicians into researchers with a capital R, but rather to give the clinician access to some nonintrusive methods for focusing clinical observations. This information can then be interpreted according to the preferred theoretical base. The advantage of the sort of measures described in this chapter is that they provide a systematic data base on which to apply the theory and may reveal aspects of the group that can get lost in the immediacy of process involvement. A discussion about psychotherapy should always begin with a firm grounding in the observed facts, before taking off into theoretical speculations.

Appendix. Selected forms

GROUP REPORT FORM

Group: _____ Date: _____ Session: _____

Therapist(s): _____

_____	_____	_____
_____		_____
_____		_____
_____	_____	_____

1. Major themes
2. Critical incidents
3. Therapist issues
4. Supervision comments
5. For next session

TARGET GOALS FORM

Name: _____ Date: _____

Please describe three goals that will be of importance for your treatment. Try to describe each goal in terms of actual personal behavior or relationship issues, not just internal feelings. Using the Rating Scale as a guide, circle the number that best describes how much that goal is bothering you at present.	RATING SCALE 0 not at all 1 a little bit 2 somewhat 3 moderately 4 quite a bit 5 a great deal 6 extremely
Goal Description	
Goal 1:	0 1 2 3 4 5 6
Goal 2:	0 1 2 3 4 5 6
Goal 3:	0 1 2 3 4 5 6

GROUP CLIMATE QUESTIONNAIRE (GCQ)

Name: _____ Group: _____ Date: _____

Read each statement carefully and try to think of the group as a whole. Using the Rating Scale as a guide, circle the number for each statement that best describes the group during today's session. Please mark only ONE answer for each statement.

RATING SCALE
0 not at all
1 a little bit
2 somewhat
3 moderately
4 quite a bit
5 a great deal
6 extremely

1. The members liked and cared about each other.	0 1 2 3 4 5 6
2. The members tried to understand why they do the things they do, tried to reason it out.	0 1 2 3 4 5 6
3. The members avoided looking at important issues going on between themselves.	0 1 2 3 4 5 6
4. The members felt what was happening was important and there was a sense of participation.	0 1 2 3 4 5 6
5. The members depended on the group leader(s) for direction.	0 1 2 3 4 5 6
6. There was friction and anger between the members.	0 1 2 3 4 5 6
7. The members were distant and withdrawn from each other.	0 1 2 3 4 5 6
8. The members challenged and confronted each other in their efforts to sort things out.	0 1 2 3 4 5 6
9. The members appeared to do things the way they thought would be acceptable to the group.	0 1 2 3 4 5 6
10. The members rejected and distrusted each other.	0 1 2 3 4 5 6
11. The members revealed sensitive personal information or feelings.	0 1 2 3 4 5 6
12. The members appeared tense and anxious.	0 1 2 3 4 5 6

Please describe briefly the event that was most personally important to you during today's session. This might be something that involved you directly, or something that happened between other members, but which made you think about yourself. Explain what it was about the event that made it important for you personally.

Source Notes

1. A review of current information regarding primate social behavior is available in *Primate Societies* (Smuts et al. 1987). An application of this material to psychotherapy groups is contained in MacKenzie and Kennedy (1989).

2. The American Group Psychotherapy Association Monograph No. 2 (Lubin and Lubin 1987) contains a listing of some 13,000 group therapy references beginning with Pratt's original articles in 1906 through to 1980. These are listed alphabetically and cross-referenced by content categories.
   Two valuable source books are available regarding original publications on group psychotherapy, many of which are difficult to obtain in the original. *Group Psychotherapy and Group Function* (Rosenbaum and Berger 1963) contains a wealth of historical articles. These make essential reading for those wanting to get a personalized flavor of the development of ideas about groups. The book also contains a selection of some papers from the early social psychology literature. The second book, *Psychoanalytic Group Dynamics: Basic Readings* (Scheidlinger 1980) is a collection of basic readings focused on papers from an analytic orientation, including several by the editor himself.

3. *Group Psychology and the Analysis of the Ego* (Freud 1921, p. 116) makes interesting reading that sheds light on the origins of some current group ideas. Freud's ideas, as well as those of G. LeBon, *The Crowd: A Study of the Popular Mind* (1896), and William McDougall, *The Group Mind* (1920), are summarized in Chapter 1 of Scheidlinger (1980). The changing views concerning the centrality of emotional expression in therapy groups are discussed by MacKenzie (1989).

4. A selection of Slavson's writings has been compiled by Mortimer Schiffer in *Dynamics of Group Psychotherapy* (Slavson 1979). Slavson was a prolific writer, and Schiffer has selected 49 articles from some 194 publications. An introduction by the editor places Slavson's work in perspective. Wolf and Schwartz's *Psychoanalysis in Groups* (1962) was a major text of its time. Fritz Redl's 1942 paper "Group Emotion and Leadership" is found in Scheidlinger (1980). Key papers by many of these group psychotherapy pioneers are found in Rosenbaum and Berger (1963).

5. Kurt Lewin's ideas are summarized in a posthumous book of collected writings edited by Cartwright, *Field Theory in Social Science* (Lewin 1951). This reveals the influence Lewin has had on both social psychology research and many aspects of group theory commonly used in therapeutic work.

   Helen Durkin provided a detailed discussion of the relevance of social psychology theories and research to clinical work in her book *The Group in Depth* (Durkin 1964). Robert F. Bales developed a three-dimensional system for describing interactional behavior: positive/negative, dominant/submissive, and task/emotion. This was presented initially in *Interaction Process Analysis* (Bales 1950) and in its most recent form in *SYMLOG—A System for the Multiple Level Observation of Groups* (Bales and Cohen 1979). The applications of Bales' ideas are well developed in a most interesting book, *Analysis of Groups* (Gibbard et al. 1974). Most of the authors are graduates from the Department of Social Relations at Harvard. Bales was a senior faculty member in that department for many years during which it was a major force in the scholarly investigation of social behavior. The book is highly recommended as a summary of the application of social psychology methodology to small groups.

   William Schutz' FIRO instrument has been widely used to measure interpersonal compatibility and as a predictor of group cohesion and outcome. The measure and its application are described in *FIRO-B: The Interpersonal Underworld* (Schutz 1966).

6. The best introduction to Bion's ideas is to read the original *Experiences in Groups and Other Papers* (1961). A commentary by M.D. Rioch (1970) may be of help. Malcolm Pines (1987) has written a thoughtful memorial piece titled "Bion: A Group Analytic Appreciation." Pines studied and worked with Foulkes in the group analytic tradition that held views at variance with Bion's approaches. Relevant analytic ideas are found in M. Klein (1946). Scheidlinger (1980) also provides a useful critique of group-as-a-whole theory.

7. A follow-up study of Tavistock patients indicated long-lasting resentment regarding the group experience and relatively poor overall outcome (Malan et al. 1976).

8. Foulkes' work is summarized in his book *Group Analytic Psychotherapy: Method and Principles* (1975).

9. These ideas about focal themes are derived from Freud's original notion about conflict involving the expression of instinctual drives, primarily of a sexual nature. Although the language of "instinct" has all but disappeared from current writings, the underlying theme of conflictual issues remains as a central tenet of psychodynamic therapy. In America, French (1954), working with Franz Alexander in Chicago, adapted these ideas for use in focused shorter-term therapy, a tradition carried into

the present by Mann and Goldman (1987), Sifneos (1987), and Davanloo (1980). In London, Ezriel (1950) (reprinted in Scheidlinger 1980) used similar concepts that were applied later by Balint et al. (1972) and Malan (1979). Horowitz (1988) expanded these approaches by incorporating the impact of cognitive schemata on relationship patterns and self-images. The main application of focal conflict theory to groups has been through a series of articles and books stemming from the University of Chicago and represented in an article by Roy Whitman and Dorothy Stock (1958) (reprinted in Scheidlinger 1980) and the book *Psychotherapy Through the Group Process* by Whitaker and Lieberman (1964). This material has been updated in a recent book by Whitaker (1985). Note that Whitaker's earlier work is published under the name Stock.

10. Since the time of its first publication in 1970, Yalom's *The Theory and Practice of Group Psychotherapy*, now in its third edition (1985), has been a leading text in the group psychotherapy field. Yalom has recently edited a section of an *American Psychiatric Association Annual Review* (Yalom 1986). There is a network of authors prominent in the group field who have been associated in various ways with Yalom, including Bond, Bloch, Lieberman, and Leszcz.

Carl Rogers' book *Client-Centered Therapy* (1951) had a profound effect on clinical practice with his ideas of "necessary and sufficient" therapist qualities. He and his senior students spawned a generation of graduate students. The theoretical basis of Rogers' ideas lies in the belief that given the right opportunity people would grow and develop (Truax et al. 1966). This optimistic stance has not withstood the test of time, at least not when applied to severely dysfunctional patients. Rogers' ideas have been to a considerable extent incorporated into the current interest in the therapeutic alliance (Docherty 1985). This work suggests that, once a minimal level of therapist interest is available, it is the contribution of the patient that plays the major role in determining the quality of the alliance (see Note 17). About the same time that Rogers was developing his theories, Jerome Frank began his pioneering work on factors common to all therapeutic approaches. Although applied to individual therapy, these quickly became incorporated into the developing interest in group therapeutic factors. His ideas are summarized in his later book *Persuasion and Healing: A Comparative Study of Psychotherapy* (Frank 1973).

In *The Interpersonal Theory of Psychiatry*, Harry Stack Sullivan (1953) developed ideas that were particularly appealing to the group therapist. Many of his ideas emerge in applied form in Yalom's text.

11. Psychodrama concepts are summarized in Moreno (1953) and gestalt techniques in Perls (1974).

12. Integrative trends are evident in Durkin (1964), Horwitz (1977a), Mullan and Rosenbaum (1978), Glatzer (1978), Scheidlinger (1983), and Yalom (1985). These developments parallel those in the individual psychotherapy literature as summarized in Beitman et al. (1989).

13. The use of object relations theory in groups as well as concepts from systems theory is discussed by Kernberg (1975). Self-psychology ideas are presented in Stone and Whitman (1977) and in Horwitz's AGPA Presidential Address (1984). The group

treatment of patients with the borderline syndrome is reviewed in Horwitz (1977b) and Stone and Gustafson (1982). A recent group text, *Psychodynamic Group Psychotherapy* (Rutan and Stone 1984), reflects a psychoanalytic psychotherapy orientation, as does the article by Alonso and Rutan (1988). General Systems Theory is applied to groups by Durkin (1981), in a multiauthored book growing out of the proceedings of the AGPA General Systems Theory interest group.

14. The literature concerning time-limited group psychotherapy is of relatively recent origin. Most of the group research literature deals with short-term groups (see Note 88), as does the inpatient group literature (see Note 76). The social psychology literature concerning group dynamics (see Note 5) as well as studies of encounter groups (Lieberman et al. 1973) and self-help groups (Lieberman and Borman 1979) also deal with brief approaches. The application of this material to clinical psychotherapy groups can be traced through the following references. Bernard and Klein (1977) and Waxer (1977) discussed emerging trends in conducting brief groups. Imber et al. (1979) described the use of a 6-session crisis group; this article contains a review of the literature concerning brief groups. Most references are from the 1970s and deal either with crisis groups or groups for acute situations such as post--myocardial infarction. Budman et al. (1980) described 15- to 20-session groups with more ambitious therapeutic goals. In particular, they accelerated the process of therapeutic work by composing groups of individuals dealing with a similar level of adult developmental tasks. This material has been updated in Budman and Gurman (1988). K.R. MacKenzie and W.J. Livesley discussed a theory of group development in the context of time-limited therapy in AGPA Monograph No. 1 (Dies and MacKenzie 1983). Goldberg et al. (1983) described 12-session groups in which the work is facilitated by the use of single-sex groups composed of members with a common focal theme. The July 1985 issue (Vol. 35, No. 3) of the *International Journal of Group Psychotherapy* has a series of articles concerning brief groups. Robert Klein and Kent Poey discussed general strategies and Robert Dies reviewed central issues regarding style of leadership. MacKenzie et al. (1986) described groups for patients with bulimia nervosa. McCallum and Piper (1988) presented a thoughtful review of critical issues in adapting analytically oriented work to brief groups. Their work is particularly interesting because, as with that of Budman, it originates in a clinical program with a strong research component. Winston et al. (1986) discussed the supposed differences between supportive and expressive therapies and provided a summary of techniques that has many similarities to the therapeutic factors discussed in this book.

Chapter 2.   The Small Group 19

15. The literature concerning the social psychology of small groups is well represented in the third edition of Cartwright and Zander's multiauthored book *Group Dynamics: Research and Theory* (1968).

16. Cohesion has been studied in a variety of ways. Piper et al. (1983) provided a review of the problems encountered in finding a satisfactory operational definition of the concept. Drescher et al. (1985) reviewed the cohesion literature. Bloch and Crouch (1985) discussed the theoretical and research literature in the context of therapeutic factors. Because cohesion entails many subjective qualities, the most satisfactory

studies stress harder data such as attendance and communication patterns. Some of the items listed as characteristic of a cohesive group are included in a recent instrument developed by Budman et al. (1987). This scoring system could be used informally in clinical settings as a way for clinicians to structure their assessment of group cohesion. Several additional ways of measuring cohesion are discussed in Chapter 16 under Process Measures. Liberman (1970) discussed behavioral strategies to reinforce cohesive behavior. The connections between cohesion and outcome are addressed by T.J. Kaul and R.L. Bednar in "Experiential Group Research: Results, Questions and Suggestions" in the *Handbook of Psychotherapy and Behavior Change* (Garfield and Bergin 1986). *Group Cohesion: Theoretical and Clinical Perspectives* by Kellerman (1981) is recommended for advanced reading. This book contains theoretical contributions regarding the importance of belonging by authors from diverse fields. It includes a particularly interesting section on evolutionary phenomena.

17. Bordin (1979) provided a thoughtful discussion of the idea of the therapeutic alliance that has served to stimulate much research activity. The section by Docherty (1985) in *Psychiatry Update: American Psychiatric Association Annual Review, Volume 4*, contains a good introduction to the concept of the therapeutic alliance. A review article by Winston et al. (1986) contains a careful definition of supportive techniques.

18. A thorough background concerning social climate is found in Moos (1974). Application to therapy groups is contained in MacKenzie (1981), MacKenzie's chapter on group climate in Dies and MacKenzie (1983), and MacKenzie et al. (1987).

19. A review of the social psychology literature concerning norms is found in Biddle (1979). MacKenzie (1979) provided an introduction to the concept of norms in therapy groups. Bond, in a chapter titled "Norm Regulation in Therapy Groups" (in Dies and MacKenzie 1983) as well as in Bond (1984), described the two-by-two matrix used in this section for considering specific normative dimensions.

20. A discussion of the effects of group size on participation can be found in Chapter 1 by Mullen in Mullen and Goethals (1987). The discussion concerning the various categories of group size is based in part on Hare (1976).

21. These ideas are explored at more length in Mullen and Goethals (1987), particularly in Chapter 2 by Goethals and Darley and in Chapter 7 by Mullen. Bandura (1986) summarized the findings of social cognition theory. Many of these same principles have been incorporated into cognitive-behavioral strategies for treating depression (Rush and Beck 1988).

Chapter 3.   The Group System. 33

22. The language of General Systems Theory now is part of the clinical vocabulary. Unfortunately, sometimes the terms are used without a serious look at their original meanings. A general introduction is provided in Durkin (1981). This multiauthored book, although sometimes a bit heavy on GST jargon, tries to take a serious look at the paradigm shift inherent in adopting a GST position.

23. Kernberg (1975) explored some of these ideas regarding the complexity of group phenomena. He uses the term *nonconcentric overlapping hierarchies* to describe the varying connections that may develop between sociocultural, group, and individual matters. The role of the therapist as a participant at all of these levels is emphasized with the potential to choose the most appropriate boundary focus.

24. The seminal early paper regarding therapeutic factors was written by Corsini and Rosenberg (1955). Yalom (1985) was instrumental in popularizing the idea of therapeutic factors and a major portion of his text is devoted to the subject. Bloch and Crouch (1985) provided a careful review of the original concepts in the light of subsequent research studies. Their book was written with the clinician in mind. A concise update of this material is found in Yalom (1986).

Chapter 4.   How Groups Develop............... 47

25. The idea of group development has a lengthy history. Tuckman (1965) provided a detailed review of the literature and proposed an integrated view. A major analysis of the literature as well as results from transcript analysis of several groups is found in Beck (1974), who identified nine stages. The first five and the last are similar in nature to those described in this book. A sixth stage deals with integration of the leader into the group, a seventh with deeper self-confrontation in a flexible group structure where role behaviors have become widely dispersed throughout the membership, and an eighth stage focuses on transfer of learning to outside situations. Saravay (1978), Lacoursiere (1980), and MacKenzie and Livesley (in Dies and MacKenzie 1983) have also contributed to the recent literature.

The one apparent exception to the usual approach is the system proposed by W.G. Bennis and H.A. Shepard in "A Theory of Group Development" (in Gibbard et al. 1974). They divided group development into two major categories labeled dependence and interdependence, each with three subphases. Although this system appears initially quite different from the one used in this book, in fact there is considerable conceptual similarity beneath the slightly different language. Bennis and Shepard appear to be describing the spiraling process by which similar themes are managed at deeper levels over time. Their thoughtful presentation makes interesting reading for one interested in the phenomena of group stages.

26. Tuckman (1965) popularized the idea of stages with the terms *forming, storming, norming, and performing*, to which others have added *adjourning*. Although these terms are catchy, the use of *norming* to describe the third stage is problematic. One of the major tasks of the storming or differentiation stage is to question group traditions that were put in place by the leader. Thus, it is the second stage that is primarily preoccupied with norming issues. In the individuation stage, which follows the results of this challenge, processes reveal a group that has now developed stronger norms.

Chapter 5.   Social Roles....................... 61

27. Early ideas regarding social roles are found in Newcombe (1950) and Slater (1955). Biddle (1979) provided a comprehensive introduction to the social psychology literature regarding social roles.

28. Beck (1974), using the term *distributed leadership*, provided a detailed description of the functional importance of role behaviors for mastering group developmental
stages. These ideas are developed in greater detail along with sociometric data in
Beck and Peters (1981). MacKenzie's chapter "The Concept of Role as a Boundary
Structure in Small Groups" (in Durkin 1981) elaborates the functional significance of
social roles. Livesley and MacKenzie (in Dies and MacKenzie 1983) applied a similar
orientation to the concept of social role with some modification of the details. There is
some discrepancy between the labels used by Beck and those used in this book. The
structural role is assumed by Beck to be the designated leader and is given a broader
role definition that includes many of the attributes of positive leadership. The sociable
role is closely related to Beck's emotional leader. The divergent role is termed the
scapegoat in Beck's system. The cautionary role is labeled the defiant member by
Beck, who stresses the challenge side of the role more than the underlying sense of
social alienation. Beck provided a particularly helpful description of this person as
managing a compromise solution to group membership by aligning with the leader in
a special relationship.

In some of the sociology literature, the assumption is made that only one
member can be a role leader. This unnecessarily restricts the use of the role concepts.
One potential liability of thinking in terms of single role leaders is that it may
encourage a subtle process of role stereotyping, which can make it difficult for the
individual so identified to try out alternative behaviors. This is in keeping with the idea
of psychological maturity being characterized by role flexibility. In clinical situations,
it is useful to think of the sum of role resources available in the total group membership.

Chapter 6. Assessment 77

29. The basic structure of the Axis II categories is coming under increasing scrutiny.
The issues are summarized in Eysenck (1987), McLemore and Brokaw (1987), Tyrer
(1988), and Widiger et al. (1988). The renewed interest in personality is relevant to the
psychotherapy literature because a dimensional conceptualization of personality fits
nicely with the idea of establishing a focus for therapeutic intervention. An expanded
view of personality organization is contained in Shapiro (1965).

30. For a review of the recent brief individual psychotherapy literature see MacKenzie
(1988). Winston et al. (1986) provided a thoughtful discussion of the boundary between supportive and expressive techniques. This literature is rapidly expanding and
makes useful reading for the therapist attempting time-limited approaches in groups.
Basic reading is provided in Malan (1979), Davanloo (1980), Strupp and Binder (1984),
Gustafson (1986), Sifneos (1987), Mann and Goldman (1987), Bauer and Kobos
(1987), and Budman and Gurman (1988). The chapter by M.P. Koss and J.N. Butcher,
"Research on Brief Psychotherapy," in Garfield and Bergin (1986) is also informative.
Ideas from these sources are applied to the assessment process discussed in the
remainder of Chapter 6.

31. Piper (1987) recently reported the use of a psychological mindedness rating
procedure. After viewing a brief videotape of a person describing a distressing situation involving close relationships, the patient is asked to explain what might be

troubling the person on the tape. The response is rated using a single-dimensional scale of psychological mindedness. The discussion in the main text is to a major extent drawn from this instrument. Piper reported a strong correlation between level of psychological mindedness using this simple technique and the likelihood that the patient will complete a course of brief group psychotherapy. Such a procedure is inherent in any assessment interview where interpersonal vignettes often form a major portion of the history. Careful attention to the manner in which these are described will yield important clues regarding the patient's capacity for psychological mindedness.

32. The technique for determining the Core Conflictual Relationship Theme is described in Luborsky's text (1984). Many of the research findings from the Penn Psychotherapy Research Project developed by Luborsky are summarized in Luborsky et al. (1988).

33. These ideas are developed by M.J. Horowitz (1987, 1988), the latter written as an introductory text for individual therapy.

34. A formal description of interpersonal therapy is found in *Interpersonal Psychotherapy of Depression* by Klerman et al. (1984). This treatment approach is particularly interesting because it was used in the large NIMH Collaborative Study of the Treatment of Depression (see Note 69).

35. The work by Budman et al. (1980) also stemmed from a research setting. His idea of composing groups according to developmental issues is an excellent application of theory to practice in a busy outpatient service setting.

Chapter 7.   Composition and Preparation 97

36. An important survey of the older literature concerning group selection criteria is found in Woods and Melnick (1979).

37. Budman and Gurman (1988) presented a model of group homogeneity based on adult developmental stages.

38. A comprehensive survey of the pretherapy preparation literature is contained in Piper and Perrault (1989). Most programs use a combination of educational methods, such as video modeling and an introductory group experience, often combined with a handout that the patient can read at leisure. The patient information material contained in this book is suitable for this purpose.

Chapter 8.   The Beginning 115

39. Bednar et al. (1974) presented a detailed rationale for the therapist to provide more structure early in a group and modify this over time. Dies, in his review chapter "Clinical Implications of Research on Leadership in Short-term Group Psychotherapy" (in Dies and MacKenzie 1983), comes to similar conclusions.

40. The question of premature terminations is addressed in Dies and Teleska (1985) and by Kaul and Bednar in Garfield and Bergin (1986). Lieberman et al. (1973) found that leaders who pressured members for early self-disclosure had higher dropout levels as did leaders who showed little involvement in the group process.

Chapter 9. Differentiation 141

41. The dominance hierarchy (MacKenzie and Kennedy 1989) is a fundamental property of primate social systems. It serves to regulate power and aggression so that they do not become destructive forces. The hierarchy is to some extent based on physical strength, but kinship support and negotiated coalitions play an important part as well. Position in the hierarchy is a major determinant of sexual access. Interestingly, dominance has not been systematically studied in therapy groups.

42. Studies of premature terminators and group casualties cite early conflict as a precipitant (Dies and Teleska 1985). This is often associated with a negative or hostile therapeutic style (Lieberman et al. 1973; Hartley et al. 1976) or a failure to develop supportive group norms (Bond in Dies and MacKenzie 1983).

43. The problems of projective mechanisms and scapegoating are expanded in Scheidlinger (1982), Horwitz (1983), and Wright et al. (1988). These phenomena are pervasive in therapy groups, and this extra reading is recommended when confronted with the need to address such issues. They are always accompanied by considerable affective arousal, and the therapist is best prepared with a solid cognitive introduction to the issues.

Chapter 10. The Working Group 159

44. The Hill Interaction Matrix (Hill 1965, 1977), one of the oldest and most widely used systems for categorizing group interaction, uses this terminology of *prework* and *work* levels. It is described in more detail in Chapter 16. The HIM has three prework categories of interaction:

Responsive—Members are responding to therapist suggestions.
Conventional—Representing social conversation about general interest topics.
Assertive—Members make argumentative or assertive statements revealing biases, beliefs, or prejudices and do not solicit or accept help from other members.

The first two of these work styles are typical of engagement stage behaviors, and the third is characteristic of the differentiation stage. The HIM has two work categories:

Speculative—There is interest in exploring interactional topics in a cooperative and task-oriented manner.
Confrontive—There is a higher level of risk taking and tension around content material usually avoided.

45. Alexander and French (1946/1980) coined the term *corrective emotional experi-ence* to refer to a type of relationship in the therapy setting in which the patient was both supported and challenged regarding areas of distortion or overreaction. Their work is commonly cited as the first major publication on brief psychotherapy. Gustafson (1986) provided a readable and stimulating overview of the development of ideas in this area.

46. The Encounter Group Study (Lieberman et al. 1973) drew attention to the impor-tance of cognitive integration of affectively powerful group experience. Dies' leader-ship chapter in Dies and MacKenzie (1983) reviews the literature in regard to the relative effectiveness of affective versus cognitive dimensions. Luborsky et al. (1988) and L.M. Horowitz (1986) demonstrated the importance of maintaining a consistent work focus for effective individual therapy.

47. The Johari Window (Luft 1970) was described by, and named after, Joseph Luft and Harry Ingram. It was initially developed for use in T-groups but can be applied just as effectively to therapy groups.

48. Jacobs (1974) provided a review of the technical dimensions of feedback. The principles involved in the feedback process are continuously operative. It is helpful for the therapist to use them knowledgeably rather than by accident.

49. The American psychologist George Kelly (1955) described in some detail the process by which the individual creates a personal view of reality. The use of Kelly's *repertory grid* technique to determine patterns of construct usage has been elabo-rated by numerous authors. An introduction to this literature can be found in Landfield and Epting (1979), Bannister and Fransella (1982), and Neimeyer and Neimeyer (1987). These ideas are now merging with the growing interest in cognitive mediating mechanisms reflected, for example, in the brief psychotherapy literature (Ryle 1979; Horowitz 1988) and in treatment of depression (Rush and Beck 1988). Recently, the *International Journal of Personal Construct Psychology* began publication (Hemi-sphere Publishing Corporation, New York).

50. The idea of critical incidents goes back a long way in the group literature. The Encounter Group Study (Lieberman et al. 1973) formalized the approach through the use of a critical incident questionnaire. A version of this in described in Chapter 16.

51. Yalom (1985) discussed this type of learning process in critical incidents as an enactment of a corrective emotional experience.

52. Ekman et al. (1972) presented a sophisticated analysis of facial behavior very much in keeping with Darwin's original observations (1872). Ekman concluded that basic affect states are "hard wired" into facial responses to form an innate communi-cation system. Plutchik (1980) and MacKenzie and Kennedy (1989) described an evolutionary perspective.

53. See Note 9 regarding the historical background to these ideas. Malan (1979) popularized the term *triangle of conflict* in his work with brief individual psychother-

apy. The discussion in the main text is derived in part from Malan's writings. Much of the current research on individual psychotherapy has incorporated similar concepts, including Benjamin (1984), Horowitz et al. (1984), Klerman et al. (1984), Luborsky (1984), Strupp and Binder (1984), and Piper et al. (1986).

54. Rutan et al. (1988) developed the idea of defenses, not as the enemies of therapeutic work, but as necessary ingredients to effective therapy.

Chapter 11.   Termination 185

55. This quote is from p. 42 in Mann and Goldman (1982/1987). These authors utilized what I have called the "Procrustean alternative" to the question of therapeutic time limits (MacKenzie 1988). All patients receive the same amount of time, in Mann's case 12 individual sessions. It is contended that this minimizes regression and ensures that the patient must deal directly with the issues of personal responsibility for change. In actual practice, patients are carefully selected for this approach; all are not forced into such time constraints. The time limit seems particularly well suited to situations in which patients are dealing with issues of autonomy, for example, student populations.

56. Budman et al. (1988) compared the results of brief individual treatment to group treatment in an outpatient sample. There was no significant difference in outcome: patients in both modalities achieved marked improvement. However, the group patients reported much less satisfaction with their treatment. Budman suggested that systematic pretherapy preparation may help this perception of having received "second-rate" therapy.

Chapter 12.   Therapist Style. 195

57. The four style dimensions of caring, meaning-attribution, executive function, and emotional stimulation have been found in many studies. They are documented particularly clearly in the Encounter Group Study (Lieberman et al. 1973). Figure 12-1 is based on data from that study. The literature concerning the effects of leader control is summarized in the chapter by Kaul and Bednar in Garfield and Bergin (1986), as well as the chapter by Dies on leadership in Dies and MacKenzie (1983). Rutan and Stone (1984) presented a series of leader style and leader focus dimensions that help to structure a discussion of leadership. Their style dimensions of activity/nonactivity and transparency/opaqueness are relevant to material in this chapter and their third style dimension of gratification/frustration is included in the discussion of interventions in Chapter 13.

58. Notes 10 and 17 introduce these topics concerning a positive and facilitating therapeutic environment.

59. Evidence is accumulating that consistent attention to a focal theme promotes greater improvement. This effect is superimposed on the benefits of a positive working alliance (Malan 1979; Marziali 1984; Piper et al. 1986; McCallum and Piper 1988).

60. Bednar et al. (1974) provided a theoretical introduction to the idea of group structuring activity. Dies (1985) discussed in detail the question of leader attitude toward controlling behavior under the provocative title "Leadership in Short-term Group Therapy: Manipulation or Facilitation?" Similar issues are raised under the heading of patient autonomy in Chapter 15.

61. Negative statements implying anger, distrust, or disengagement from the therapist have been found to have antitherapeutic effects in numerous studies (Dies and Cohen 1976; Lieberman et al. 1973). Even negative interaction between cotherapists can be counterproductive (Dies et al. 1979). See also Note 81.

62. A major review of the therapist self-disclosure literature is found in Dies (1977), with an updated summary in Dies and MacKenzie (1983). Dies concluded that self-disclosure by the therapist becomes less appropriate as the patient population becomes more psychologically impaired, and that selective self-disclosure may become more appropriate as a group moves into more advanced working stages.

Chapter 13.   The Therapeutic Encounter. 209

63. The reader is referred to a discussion of these matters in West and Livesley (1986). The same issue of that journal includes critical commentaries by several prominent group therapists regarding their article. The principal area of disagreement centers on the relative importance of the personal encounter with the therapist. This is a real experience that is not "as if" in nature. Therapists from a Rogerian or self-psychology tradition place greater emphasis on this aspect of the therapeutic relationship.

64. There is considerable interest in current psychotherapy research regarding the matter of intervention style and accuracy. One part of this work uses some way of identifying a focal theme and then measuring how consistently the therapist attends to this theme. Some of the major contributors include Benjamin (1984) from the University of Utah; L.M. Horowitz (1986) from Stanford; M.J. Horowitz (1988) from Langley Porter, San Francisco; Luborsky et al. (1988) from the University of Pennsylvania project; Piper (1988) from the University of Alberta; Strupp and Binder (1984) from the Vanderbilt project; and Winston (1988) from Beth Israel, New York. In Chapter 6, some techniques developed in these studies were introduced.

65. The effect of clarification versus confrontation techniques in terms of their ability to promote effective introspective work is reported by Winston (1988). Scheidlinger (1987) provided a thoughtful clinical discussion of how the therapist might approach the use of interpretations. Winston et al. (1986) discussed the difference between supportive and expressive techniques. Confrontation methods would generally be classed as expressive. However, the discussion in the main text concerning the effective use of clarification indicates how the boundary between the two may become blurred.

66. An article by Stone and Gustafson (1982) provides a good beginning reference for the treatment of severe character pathology. It is one of a series of articles on this topic in that particular issue of the *International Journal of Group Psychotherapy*.

Rutan and Stone's text (1984) also reflects a psychoanalytic orientation. Articles by Kernberg (1975), Glatzer (1978), Horwitz (1977a, 1977b, 1983, 1984), Scheidlinger (1987), Alonso and Rutan (1988), and McCallum and Piper (1988) trace the development of analytic ideas in group therapy.

67. The literature concerning negative effects has been summarized by Strupp et al. (1977), Sachs (1983), Dies and Teleska (1985), and Kaul and Bednar in Garfield and Bergin (1986).

Chapter 14.   Group Programs. 225

68. The outcome literature is surveyed in Smith et al. (1980); Shapiro and Shapiro (1982); Steinbrueck et al. (1983); Docherty (1985); Garfield and Bergin (1986) (see particularly chapters by Kaul and Bednar; Koss and Butcher; Lambert et al.).

69. The NIMH Collaborative Study of the Treatment of Depression provides one of the larger attempts at comparing different approaches using controlled treatment conditions for cognitive therapy, interpersonal psychotherapy, antidepressants (imipramine), and a control clinical management. Preliminary results suggest that all three treatment conditions achieved significant improvement. In the most severely depressed patients, the interpersonal psychotherapy and imipramine produced similar effects. These results are somewhat surprising, and further details of the study will be of value in clarifying specific predictors of therapeutic response (Weissman et al. 1987).

70. Toseland and Siporin (1986) reviewed 32 controlled studies that compared individual and group treatments. These spanned a wide variety of theoretical orientations and patient populations. Group treatment was found as effective as individual treatment in 75% of these, and more effective in 25%. At the same time, the authors correctly pointed out that many of the studies, although using randomization techniques, were not methodologically entirely satisfactory. Several recent investigations have specifically compared individual and group approaches (Pilkonis et al. 1984; Piper et al. 1984; Budman et al. 1988).

71. The Budman study referenced in Note 70 included patient satisfaction measures as well as health-care utilization statistics, which make it particularly relevant to clinical settings.

72. Phillips (1987) combined service statistics from a wide variety of outpatient treatment settings to produce the curve shown in Figure 14-1. Technically this is a negative Poisson distribution curve in which the mean equals the variance. The shape of the curve therefore remains constant, although the actual mean number of sessions may vary across settings.

73. Howard et al. (1986) pooled data from 15 sources involving over 2400 patients to estimate the rate of symptomatic improvement. It is important to underline the point that early improvement occurred whether or not the actual treatment course was planned to be brief or longer term. The research literature is clear enough about the

pace of change that briefer modalities should be considered as the preferred initial approach for all patients except those with major contraindications.

74. The handful of studies investigating the effect of coleadership on treatment outcome are summarized by Dies' leadership chapter in Dies and MacKenzie (1983). Two studies are particularly relevant to clinical work (Dies et al. 1979; Piper et al. 1979).

75. Rutan and Alonso (1982) and Caligor et al. (1984) discussed the implications of concurrent therapy in analytically oriented psychotherapy.

76. A more detailed introduction to the specialized nature of inpatient groups is provided in the following sources. Maxmen (1984) described a pragmatic approach well suited for most short-stay inpatient units. M. Leszcz in Yalom (1986) bases his discussion on a careful review of the literature that emphasizes group, patient, milieu, and leadership factors. Contrasting models of inpatient group therapy are found in a special section of *Hospital and Community Psychiatry* (Vol. 39, May 1988) in which Beeber discussed a systems and group developmental perspective, Brabender a private psychiatric hospital setting, and Kanas an approach for the schizophrenic inpatient. Greater emphasis on psychodynamic principles is found in Kibel (1981) and in a book by Rice and Rutan (1987). Yalom (1983) also wrote a book devoted to inpatient groups.

77. J. Bancroft, in Bloch (1986), presented a succinct synopsis of crisis intervention goals and techniques.

78. Bloch (1986) provided a description of a similar approach to long-term follow-up in his useful small book on the psychotherapies. Kanas (1986) reviewed the literature regarding controlled studies of group therapy for schizophrenic patients.

79. Lieberman and Borman (1979) gave a detailed description of types of self-help groups and the therapeutic mechanisms characteristic of each.

Chapter 15.   Ethics and Supervision 245

80. Formal guidelines for the psychiatrist are found in "The Principles of Medical Ethics With Annotations Especially Applicable to Psychiatry" developed by the Ethics Committee of the American Psychiatric Association (1985). Similar guidelines are contained in the ethics statement of other professional societies. An extended discussion of ethical topics is found in Lakin (1988).

81. Harmful therapist attitudes have been described by Strupp and Lane (1988).

82. The first major publication concerning the use of video technology in psychotherapy was by Berger (1970). Ian Alger's "Audiovisual Review" column in *Hospital and Community Psychiatry* discusses new material. For the beginning therapist, the acquisition of basic skills can be accelerated through the use of audio and video recordings. This practice may also lead to an exploration of the internal responses of

the therapist. However, it is easy, though not inevitable, for the focus on specific skills to get in the way of understanding the experience the new therapist is having and the personal reactions that may be occurring. These issues are reviewed in the context of the idea of confidentiality in Betcher and Zinberg (1988).

83. Some of these ideas have been adopted from Scott Rutan's 1987 Keynote Address to the Canadian Group Psychotherapy Association.

84. Lakin (1988) provided an extended discussion of ethical issues and psychotherapy.

85. The material in this book is written from the standpoint of the supervisee, whereas most of the available literature is directed toward the supervisor. Both parties might enjoy Alonso's book *The Quiet Profession: Supervisors of Psychotherapy* (1985), which deals sensitively with many aspects of the supervision process.

86. The formal requirements for membership in the American Group Psychotherapy Association, as well as an outline developed by the AGPA Training Committee, can be obtained from the American Group Psychotherapy Association, 25 East 21st Street, New York, NY 10010. Tel.: 212–477–2677.

87. Salvendy (1980) discussed a number of training issues, including the usefulness of an experience as the member of a therapy group.

Chapter 16.   Records and Measures 261

88. Throughout this book, reference has been made to advances in the clinical investigation of individual psychotherapy. This material is not commonly integrated into a discussion of group therapy despite its obvious relevance. A good review of current issues is found in *The Handbook of Psychotherapy and Behavior Change*, edited by Garfield and Bergin (1986). Relevant articles are also found in special psychotherapy research issues of the *American Psychologist* and the *Journal of Consulting and Clinical Psychology*, both published in February 1986. Parloff et al. (1986) offered further commentary and Piper (1988) discussed important research questions.

A valuable collection of group research articles is available in a volume edited by Roback et al. (1979). These are classic articles drawn from many diverse and difficult-to-locate sources. They represent a good survey of the field into the early 1970s after which it is easier to locate material through data base searches. Frequent reference has been made to the Encounter Group Study by Lieberman et al. (1973) because it represents one of the more comprehensive investigations of small-group functioning. Discussion of research design for investigations regarding group studies is found in Burlingame et al. (1984).

89. In AGPA Monograph No. 1 (Dies and MacKenzie 1983), Dies provided a detailed introduction to the use of structured measures in clinical settings.

90. The material concerning change measures is adapted in part from Waskow and

Parloff (1975), MacKenzie and Dies (1981), and MacKenzie and Livesley (1986). Lambert et al. in Garfield and Bergin (1986) presented a comprehensive discussion of the complexities of measuring change over time.

91. The usual method for assigning social class is the Index of Social Status developed by Hollingshead (1975).

92. Mumford et al. (1984) reviewed the evidence for a decrease in medical service utilization after psychiatric treatment. Recent data relating specifically to group programs are found in Budman et al. (1988).

93. The SCL-90-R can be obtained from Clinical Psychometric Research, Box 425, Riderwood, MD 21139.

94. The Social Adjustment Scale can be obtained from Yale University School of Medicine, Department of Psychiatry, Depression Research Unit, 904 Howard Avenue, Suite #2A, New Haven, CT 06519.

95. The Global Assessment of Functioning Form is found in the *Diagnostic and Statistical Manual of Mental Disorders, Third Edition, Revised* (DSM-III-R) (1987), published by the American Psychiatric Association, Washington, DC.

96. An orientation to SASB is found in Benjamin (1974). The details of the SASB system are included here with some trepidation, because this is not designed as a research book. However, there are some advantages to the use of a systematic method for describing interactions. The SASB method comes from a lengthy research tradition concerned with dimensions of behavior (Kiesler 1983; Tyrer 1988). In my own experience as a supervisor, I have found that SASB diagrams provide a useful orienting perspective on the processes of assessment and therapy.

The SASB system may be used in several different ways. It can be applied in a global, clinical fashion to describe a person's interactional style. It can be used in detailed research applications to rate transcripts sentence by sentence. Or it may be used in a questionnaire format for patient self-report. In the main text, a simplified version of SASB is used. It consists only of the two principal axes: positive/negative affiliation and independence/interdependence. Use of this two-dimensional space can be quite useful in plotting the relationships among interpersonal events or themes. However, it does not really do justice to the full elaboration of the SASB system. That requires the addition of another level—the focus. To fully apply SASB to a specific interactional sequence, three sequential decisions are made:

Relationship focus. Three possibilities are provided. The first focus is that of "acting on" the other. For the grammatically inclined, this involves a transitive verb of doing something to another. For example, trying to understand (the other), nurturing, blaming, or ignoring (the other). The second focus is the self "reacting to" what someone else is doing. This is an intransitive verb that does not require an object. (I am) disclosing, trusting, protesting, or withdrawing are reactive states. The third focus is introspective, that is, doing something to the self. This would include such items as trying to understand self, nurturing self (these two are related to self-esteem), blaming self, or neglecting self. The choice of focus is usually quite evident.

Affiliation rating. At one end this is characterized by joy, love, and connecting, and at the other by anger, rejecting, and protesting. This positive/negative rating is easily and reliably made.

Interdependence rating. A judgment regarding this dimension is not as easy to make. At one end is an autonomous or independent state, and at the other an enmeshed or interdependent one. The focus decision made in step 1 now effects the ratings. If a transitive "acting on the other" focus was chosen, then the scale ranges from controlling (the other) to giving the other autonomy. If the intransitive "reacting to other" focus applies, then the scale ranges from submitting (to the other) to self-assertion. If the transaction was an introjection, the vertical scale ranges from controlling self to letting the self go. In making these ratings, one may encounter a discrepancy between the verbal content and the interpersonal process. For example, assertion must be differentiated from control, and attempts to understand from nurturance.

With some practice, these three decisions can be made quite quickly. The system of descriptors is shown in the following figure. It simply reflects three circles, one for each focus, based on the dimensions of affiliation and interdependence. The circular space described by the two axes is broken down into eight descriptors for each of the three foci. This produces a total of 16 interpersonal dimensions and 8 introspective items.

Think of a particular patient and work your way through the three circles to find the most appropriate location. It is easiest to think of each circle having four quadrants, representing high or low scores on each dimension. Now think of a particular interaction between two people and consider where each participant resides in the SASB space. Usually, complementary placements are found. For example, one person might be found in the lower-right quadrant of the transitive space (nurturing and protecting), whereas the other is found in the same quadrant of the intransitive space (trusting and relying on).

This system has attracted interest in the psychotherapy research literature as a descriptive system for categorizing behavior. It is compatible with a long history of dimensional ideas about interpersonal function. SASB presents these ideas in a very usable manner that has a comfortable feel for the clinician. Further information can be obtained from the author: Dr. Lorna Benjamin, Department of Psychology, University of Utah, Salt Lake City, UT 84112.

97. Process measures are reviewed in MacKenzie and Livesley (1986) and in Fuhriman and Packard (1986). Kaul and Bednar in Garfield and Bergin (1986) presented an overview of the current state of group research.

98. The Group Climate Questionnaire is described in MacKenzie (1981), and an applied example is provided in a study of training groups (MacKenzie et al. 1987). The factor structure has been replicated on several different populations. Results may be reported as raw scores or normative scores based on a sample of nonpsychotic outpatient groups.

SASB CLUSTER TERMINOLOGY
In terms of our relationship, I am:

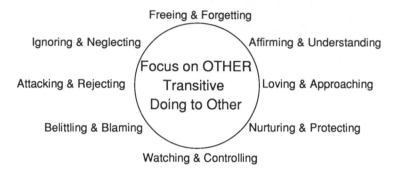

Freeing & Forgetting

Ignoring & Neglecting

Affirming & Understanding

Focus on OTHER
Transitive
Doing to Other

Attacking & Rejecting

Loving & Approaching

Belittling & Blaming

Nurturing & Protecting

Watching & Controlling

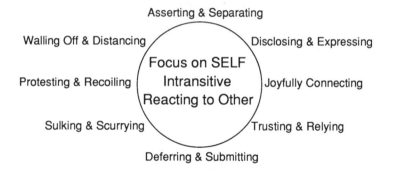

Asserting & Separating

Walling Off & Distancing

Disclosing & Expressing

Focus on SELF
Intransitive
Reacting to Other

Protesting & Recoiling

Joyfully Connecting

Sulking & Scurrying

Trusting & Relying

Deferring & Submitting

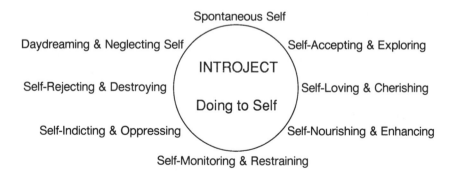

Spontaneous Self

Daydreaming & Neglecting Self

Self-Accepting & Exploring

INTROJECT

Doing to Self

Self-Rejecting & Destroying

Self-Loving & Cherishing

Self-Indicting & Oppressing

Self-Nourishing & Enhancing

Self-Monitoring & Restraining

Structural Analysis of Social Behavior (SASB) cluster version.

1. Calculate T-scores for EACH item using the following formulas (x = item raw score). Round results to nearest integer.

       Item 1: $50 + [(x - 3.77)/0.117]$
       Item 2: $50 + [(x - 3.70)/0.124]$
       Item 3: $50 + [(x - 2.06)/0.149]$
       Item 4: $50 + [(x - 3.90)/0.139]$
       Item 5: $50 + [(x - 2.52)/0.151]$
       Item 6: $50 + [(x - 1.83)/0.146]$
       Item 7: $50 + [(x - 1.75)/0.131]$
       Item 8: $50 + [(x - 3.28)/0.148]$
       Item 9: $50 + [(x - 2.30)/0.141]$
       Item 10: $50 + [(x - 1.13)/0.121]$
       Item 11: $50 + [(x\ \ 3.41)/0.157]$
       Item 12: $50 + [(x - 2.24)/0.146]$

2. Scale scores are calculated by taking the mean of the relevant items, then dividing by the actual number used. If more than four items are missing, the test is invalid. Round scale results to the nearest integer.

ENGAGED (a positive, working climate): $(1 + 2 + 4 + 8 + 11)/5$

CONFLICT (anger and rejection): $(6 + 7 + 10 + 12)/4$

AVOIDING (personal responsibility for group work): $(3 + 5 + 9)/3$

99. The Group Environment Scale, as well as a theoretical introduction to the concept of social climate, is found in Moos (1974).

100. MacKenzie (1987) discussed the use of critical incidents to assess the presence of therapeutic factors. A detailed discussion of ways to rate critical incidents is found in Bloch and Crouch (1985).

101. The Hill Interaction Matrix is described by Hill (1965, 1977). See also Note 44.

102. This quote by Morris Parloff (1980), a long-standing leader in the field of psychotherapy research, is from Dies' introductory chapter "Bridging the Gap Between Research and Practice in Group Psychotherapy" in the first AGPA Monograph (Dies and MacKenzie 1983).

Selected References

Alexander F, French TM: Psychoanalytic Therapy: Principles and Application (1946). Lincoln, NE, University of Nebraska Press, 1980

Alonso A: The Quiet Profession: Supervisors of Psychotherapy. New York, Macmillan, 1985

Alonso A, Rutan JS: The experience of shame and the restoration of self-respect in group therapy. Int J Group Psychother 38:3–14, 1988

American Psychiatric Association: The Principles of Medical Ethics With Annotations Especially Applicable to Psychiatry. Washington, DC, American Psychiatric Association, 1985

American Psychiatric Association: Diagnostic and Statistical Manual of Mental Disorders, Third Edition, Revised. Washington, DC, American Psychiatric Association, 1987

Bales RF: Interaction Process Analysis. Cambridge, MA, Addison-Wesley, 1950

Bales RF, Cohen SP: SYMLOG—A System for the Multiple Level Observation of Groups. New York, Free Press, 1979

Balint M, Ornstein PH, Balint E: Focal Psychotherapy. London, Tavistock, 1972

Bandura A: Social Foundations of Thought and Action: A Social Cognitive Theory. Englewood Cliffs, NJ, Prentice-Hall, 1986

Bannister D, Fransella F: Inquiring Man: The Psychology of Personal Constructs, 2nd Edition. Malabar, FL, Krieger, 1982

Bauer GP, Kobos JC: Brief Therapy: Short-term Psychodynamic Intervention. Northvale, NJ, Aronson, 1987

Beck AP: Phases in the development of structure in therapy and encounter groups, in Innovations in Client-Centered Therapy. Edited by Wexler DA, Rice LN. New York, Wiley, 1974

Beck AP, Peters L: The research evidence for distributed leadership in therapy groups. Int J Group Psychother 31:43–71, 1981

Bednar RL, Melnick J, Kaul TJ: Risk, responsibility, and structure: a conceptual framework for initiating group counselling and psychotherapy. Journal of Counselling Psychology 21:31–37, 1974

Beeber AR: A systems model for short-term, open-ended group therapy. Hosp Community Psychiatry 39:537–542, 1988

Beitman BD, Goldfried MR, Norcross JC: The movement toward integrating the psychotherapies. Am J Psychiatry 146:138–147, 1989

Benjamin LS: Structural analysis of social behavior. Psychol Rev 81:392–425, 1974

Benjamin LS: Principles of prediction using Structural Analysis of Social Behavior, in Personality and the Prediction of Behavior. Edited by Zucker RA, Aronoff J, Rabin AJ. New York, Academic Press, 1984

Berger MM: Videotape Techniques in Psychiatric Training and Treatment. New York, Brunner/Mazel, 1970

Bernard HS, Klein RH: Some perspectives on time-limited group psychotherapy. Compr Psychiatry 18:579–584, 1977

Betcher RW, Zinberg NE: Supervision and privacy in psychotherapy training. Am J Psychiatry 145:796–803, 1988

Biddle BJ: Role Theory: Expectations, Identities and Behaviors. New York, Academic Press, 1979

Bion WR: Experiences in Groups and Other Papers. New York, Basic Books, 1961

Bloch S: An Introduction to the Psychotherapies. Oxford, Oxford University Press, 1986

Bloch S, Crouch E: Therapeutic Factors in Group Psychotherapy. Oxford, Oxford University Press, 1985

Bond GR: Positive and negative norm regulation and their relationship to therapy group size. Group 8:35–44, 1984

Bordin ES: The generalizability of the psychoanalytic concept of the working alliance. Psychotherapy: Theory, Research and Practice 16:252–260, 1979

Brabender V: A closed model of short-term inpatient group psychotherapy. Hosp Community Psychiatry 39:542–545, 1988

Budman SH, Gurman AS: Theory and Practice of Brief Therapy. New York, Guilford Press, 1988

Budman SH, Bennett MJ, Wisnecki MJ: Short-term group psychotherapy: an adult developmental model. Int J Group Psychother 30:63–76, 1980

Budman SH, Demby A, Feldstein M, et al: Preliminary findings on a new instrument to measure cohesion in group psychotherapy. Int J Group Psychother 37:75–94, 1987

Budman SH, Demby A, Redondo JP, et al: Comparative outcome in time-limited individual and group psychotherapy. Int J Group Psychother 38:63–86, 1988

Burlingame G, Fuhriman A, Drescher S: Scientific inquiry into small group process. Small Group Behavior 5:440–476, 1984

Caligor J, Fieldsteel ND, Brok AJ: Individual and Group Therapy: Combining Psychoanalytic Techniques. New York, Basic Books, 1984

Cartwright D, Zander A: Group Dynamics: Research and Theory, 3rd Edition. New York, Harper and Row, 1968

Corsini R, Rosenberg B: Mechanisms of group psychotherapy: processes and dynamics. Journal of Abnormal and Social Psychology 51:406–411, 1955

Cramer-Azima FJ, Richmond LH: Adolescent group psychotherapy (AGPA Monograph No 4). Madison, CT, International Universities Press, 1989

Darwin C: The Expression of Emotions in Man and Animals. London, John Murray, 1872

Davanloo H (ed): Short-term Dynamic Psychotherapy. New York, Aronson, 1980

Dies RR: Group therapist transparency: a critique of theory and research. Int J Group Psychother 27:177–200, 1977

Dies RR: Leadership in short-term group therapy: manipulation or facilitation? Int J Group Psychother 35:435–455, 1985

Dies RR, Cohen L: Content considerations in group therapist self-disclosure. Int J Group Psychother 26:71–88, 1976

Dies RR, MacKenzie KR (eds): Advances in group psychotherapy: integrating research and practice (AGPA Monograph No 1). New York, International Universities Press, 1983

Dies RR, Teleska PA: Negative outcome in group psychotherapy, in Negative Outcome in Psychotherapy and What to Do About It. Edited by Mays DT, Franks CM. New York, Springer, 1985

Dies RR, Mallet J, Johnson F: Openness in the coleader relationship: its effect on group process and outcome. Small Group Behavior 10:523–546, 1979

Docherty JP (section ed): Section V: The therapeutic alliance and treatment outcome, in Psychiatry Update: American Psychiatric Association Annual Review, Vol 4. Edited by Hales RE, Frances AJ. Washington, DC, American Psychiatric Press, 1985

Drescher S, Burlingame G, Fuhriman A: Cohesion: an odyssey in empirical understanding. Small Group Behavior 16:3–30, 1985

Durkin HE: The Group in Depth. New York, International Universities Press, 1964

Durkin JE: Living Groups: Group Psychotherapy and General System Theory. New York, Brunner/Mazel, 1981

Ekman P, Friesen WV, Ellsworth P: Emotion in the Human Face. New York, Pergamon, 1972

Eysenck HJ: The definition of personality disorders and the criteria appropriate for their description. Journal of Personality Disorders 1:211–219, 1987

Foulkes SH: Group Analytic Psychotherapy: Method and Principles. London, Gordon & Breach, 1975

Frank JD: Persuasion and Healing: A Comparative Study of Psychotherapy. Baltimore, MD, Johns Hopkins University Press, 1973

French TM: The Integration of Behavior: The Integrative Process in Dreams. Chicago, IL, University of Chicago Press, 1954

Freud S: Group Psychology and the Analysis of the Ego (1921). Standard Edition, Vol 18. London, Hogarth Press, 1955, pp 67–143

Fuhriman A, Packard T: Group process instruments: therapeutic themes and issues. Int J Group Psychother 36:399–425, 1986

Garfield SL, Bergin AE (eds): Handbook of Psychotherapy and Behavior Change. New York, Wiley, 1986

Gibbard GS, Hartman JJ, Mann RD (eds): Analysis of Groups. San Francisco, CA, Jossey-Bass, 1974

Glatzer HT: The working alliance in analytic group psychotherapy. Int J Group Psychother 28:147–161, 1978

Goldberg DA, Schuyler WR, Bransfield D, et al: Focal group psychotherapy: a dynamic approach. Int J Group Psychother 33:413–431, 1983

Gustafson JP: The Complex Secret of Brief Psychotherapy. New York, Norton, 1986

Hare AP: Handbook of Small Group Research, 2nd Edition. New York, Free Press, 1976

Hartley D, Roback HB, Abramowitz SI: Deterioration effects in encounter groups. Am Psychol 31:247–255, 1976

Hill WF: Hill Interaction Matrix Manual and Supplement, Revised Edition. Los Angeles, University of Southern California, Youth Studies Center, 1965

Hill WF: Hill Interaction Matrix (HIM): the conceptual framework, derived rating scales, and an updated bibliography. Small Group Behavior 8:251–268, 1977

Hollingshead AB: Four Factor Index of Social Status. New Haven, CT, Yale University, Department of Sociology, 1975

Horowitz LM, Vitkus J: The interpersonal basis of psychiatric symptoms. Clinical Psychological Review 6:443–469, 1986

Horowitz MJ: States of Mind: Analysis of Change in Psychotherapy, 2nd Edition. New York, Plenum, 1987

Horowitz MJ: Introduction to Psychodynamics: A New Synthesis. New York, Basic Books, 1988

Horowitz MJ, Marmar C, Krupnick J, et al: Personality Styles and Brief Psychotherapy. New York, Guilford Press, 1984

Horwitz L: A group-centered approach to group psychotherapy. Int J Group Psychother 27:423–439, 1977a

Horwitz L: Group psychotherapy of the borderline patient, in Borderline Personality Disorders. Edited by Hartocollis P. New York, International Universities Press, 1977b

Horwitz L: Projective identification in dyads and groups. Int J Group Psychother 33:319–330, 1983

Horwitz L: Presidential Address: The self in groups. Int J Group Psychother 34:519–540, 1984

Howard KI, Kopta SM, Krause MS, et al: The dose-effect relationship in psychotherapy. Am Psychol 41:159–164, 1986

Imber SD, Lewis PM, Loiselle RH: Uses and abuses of the brief intervention group. Int J Group Psychother 29:39–49, 1979

Jacobs A: The use of feedback in groups, in The Group as Agent of Change. Edited by Jacobs A, Spradlin W. New York, Behavioral Publications, 1974

Kanas N: Group therapy with schizophrenics: a review of controlled studies. Int J Group Psychother 36:339–351, 1986

Kanas N: Therapy group for schizophrenic patients on acute care units. Hosp Community Psychiatry 39:546–549, 1988

Kellerman H: Group Cohesion: Theoretical and Clinical Perspectives. New York, Grune and Stratton, 1981

Kelly GA: The Psychology of Personal Constructs. New York, Norton, 1955

Kernberg O: A systems approach to priority setting of interventions in groups. Int J Group Psychother 25:251–275, 1975

Kibel HD: A conceptual model for short-term inpatient group psychotherapy. Am J Psychiatry 138:74–80, 1981

Kiesler DJ: The 1982 interpersonal circle: a taxonomy for complementarity in human transactions. Psychol Rev 90:185–214, 1983

Klein M: Notes on some schizoid mechanisms. Int J Psychoanal 27:99–110, 1946

Klein RH: Some principles of short-term group therapy. Int J Group Psychother 35:309–329, 1985

Klerman GL, Weissman MM, Rounsaville BJ, et al: Interpersonal Psychotherapy of Depression. New York, Basic Books, 1984

Lacoursiere R: The Life Cycle of Groups: Group Developmental Stage Theory. New York, Human Sciences Press, 1980

Lakin M: Ethical Issues in the Psychotherapies. New York, Oxford University Press, 1988

Landfield AW, Epting FR: Personal Construct Psychology: Clinical and Personality Assessment. New York, Human Sciences Press, 1979

Lewin K: Field Theory in Social Science. New York, Harper, 1951

Liberman RA: A behavioral approach to group dynamics, 1: reinforcement and prompting of cohesion in group therapy. Behavior Therapy 1:141–175, 1970

Lieberman MA, Borman LD: Self-help Groups for Coping With Crisis. San Francisco, CA, Jossey-Bass, 1979

Lieberman MA, Yalom ID, Miles MB: Encounter Groups: First Facts. New York, Basic Books, 1973

Lubin B, Lubin AW: Comprehensive index of group psychotherapy writings (AGPA Monograph No 2). Madison, CT, International Universities Press, 1987

Luborsky L: Principles of Psychoanalytic Psychotherapy: A Manual for Supportive-Expressive Treatment. New York, Basic Books, 1984

Luborsky L, Crits-Christoph P, Mintz J, et al: Who Will Benefit From Psychotherapy? New York, Basic Books, 1988

Luft J: Group Processes: An Introduction to Group Dynamics. Palo Alto, CA, National Press, 1970

McCallum M, Piper WE: Psychoanalytically oriented short-term groups for outpatients: unsettled issues. Group 12:21–32, 1988

MacKenzie KR: Groups norms: importance and measurement. Int J Group Psychother 29:471–480, 1979

MacKenzie KR: Measurement of group climate. Int J Group Psychother 31:287–295, 1981

MacKenzie KR: Therapeutic factors in group psychotherapy: a contemporary view. Group 11:26–34, 1987

MacKenzie KR: Recent developments in brief psychotherapy. Hosp Community Psychiatry 39:742–752, 1988

MacKenzie KR: The changing role of emotion in group psychotherapy, in Emotions and Psychopathology. Edited by Plutchik R, Kellerman H. (Fourth volume in the series "Emotion: Theory, Research and Experience") New York, Academic Press, 1989

MacKenzie KR, Dies RR: CORE battery (Clinical Outcome Results) (Monograph sponsored by AGPA Research Committee). New York, American Group Psychotherapy Association, 1981

MacKenzie KR, Kennedy JW: Primate ethology and group dynamics, in Expanding World of Group Psychotherapy: Essays in Honor of Saul Scheidlinger. Edited by Tuttman S. New York, International Universities Press, 1989

MacKenzie KR, Livesley WJ: Outcome and process measures in brief group psychotherapy. Psychiatric Annals 16:715–720, 1986

MacKenzie KR, Livesley WJ, Coleman M, et al: Short-term group psychotherapy for bulimia nervosa. Psychiatric Annals 16:699–708, 1986

MacKenzie KR, Dies RR, Stone W, et al: An analysis of AGPA Institute groups. Int J Group Psychother 37:55–74, 1987

McLemore CW, Brokaw DW: Personality disorders as dysfunctional interpersonal behavior. Journal of Personality Disorders 1:270–285, 1987

MacLennan BW, Saul S, Weiner MB (eds): Group psychotherapies for the elderly (AGPA Monograph No 5). Madison, CT, International Universities Press, 1988

Malan DH: Individual Psychotherapy and the Science of Psychodynamics, 2nd Edition. London, Butterworth, 1979

Malan DH, Balfour FHG, Hood VG, et al: Group psychotherapy: a long term followup study. Arch Gen Psychiatry 33:1303–1315, 1976

Mann J, Goldman R: A Casebook in Time-Limited Psychotherapy (1982). Washington, DC, American Psychiatric Press, 1987

Marziali E: Prediction of outcome of brief psychotherapy from therapists' interpretive interventions. Arch Gen Psychiatry 41: 301–304, 1984

Maxmen JS: Helping patients survive theories: the practice of an educative model. Int J Group Psychother 34:355-368, 1984

Moos RH: Evaluating Treatment Environments. New York, Wiley, 1974

Moreno JL: Who Shall Survive? New York, Beacon House, 1953

Mullan H, Rosenbaum M: Group Psychotherapy: Theory and Practice, 2nd Edition. New York, Free Press, 1978

Mullen B, Goethals GR: Theories of Group Behavior. New York, Springer-Verlag, 1987

Mumford E, Schlesinger HJ, Glass GV, et al: A new look at evidence about reduced cost of medical utilization following mental health treatment. Am J Psychiatry 141:1145–1158, 1984

Neimeyer RA, Neimeyer GJ (eds): Personal Construct Therapy Casebook. New York, Springer, 1987

Newcombe TM: Role behaviors in the study of individual personality and of groups. J Pers 18:273-289, 1950

Parloff MB: Psychotherapy and research: an anclitic depression. Psychiatry 43:279–293, 1980

Parloff MB, London P, Wolfe B: Individual psychotherapy and behavior change. Annu Rev Psychol 37:321–349, 1986

Perls F: The Gestalt Approach and Eye Witness to Therapy. Ben Lomond, CA, Science and Behavior Books, 1974

Phillips EL: The ubiquitous decay curve: delivery similarities in psychotherapy, medicine and addiction. Professional Psychology: Research and Practice 18:650–652, 1987

Pilkonis PA, Imber SD, Lewis P, et al: A comparative outcome study of individual, group, and conjoint psychotherapy. Arch Gen Psychiatry 41:431–437, 1984

Pines M: Bion: a group-analytic appreciation. Group Analysis 20:251–262, 1987

Piper WE: Assessment of psychological mindedness. Paper presented at the meeting of the Society for Psychotherapy Research, Ulm, West Germany, 1987

Piper WE: Psychotherapy research in the 1980's: defining areas of consensus and controversy. Hosp Community Psychiatry 39:1055–1063, 1988

Piper WE, Perrault EL: Pretherapy preparation for group members. Int J Group Psychother 39:17–34, 1989

Piper WE, Doan BD, Edwards EM, et al: Cotherapy behavior, group therapy process, and treatment outcome. J Consult Clin Psychol 47:1081–1089, 1979

Piper WE, Marrache M, Lacroix R, et al: Cohesion as a basic bond in groups. Human Relations 36:93-108, 1983

Piper WE, Debbane EG, Bienvenu JP, et al: A comparative study of four forms of psychotherapy. J Consult Clin Psychol 52:268–279, 1984

Piper WE, Debbane EG, Bienvenu JP, et al: Relationships between the focus of therapist interpretations and outcome in short-term individual psychotherapy. Br J Med Psychol 59:1–11, 1986

Plutchik R: Emotion: A Psychoevolutionary Synthesis. New York, Harper and Row, 1980

Poey K: Guidelines for the practice of brief, dynamic group therapy. Int J Group Psychother 35:331–354, 1985

Rice CA, Rutan JS: Inpatient Group Psychotherapy: A Dynamic Perspective. New York, Macmillan, 1987

Riester AE, Kraft IA: Child group psychotherapy (AGPA Monograph No 3). Madison, CT, International Universities Press, 1986

Rioch MD: The work of Wilfred Bion on groups. Psychiatry 33:56–66, 1970

Roback HB, Abramowitz SI, Strassberg DS: Group Psychotherapy Research: Commentaries and Selected Readings. Huntington, NY, Krieger, 1979

Rogers CR: Client-Centered Therapy. London, Constable, 1951

Rosenbaum M, Berger M: Group Psychotherapy and Group Function. New York, Basic Books, 1963

Rush AJ, Beck AT (section eds): Section V: Cognitive therapy, in American Psychiatric Press Review of Psychiatry, Vol 7. Edited by Frances AJ, Hales RE. Washington, DC, American Psychiatric Press, 1988

Rutan JS: The faith of the group therapist. Keynote Address at the annual meeting of the Canadian Group Psychotherapy Association, Mount Tremblant, Quebec, 1987

Rutan JS, Alonso A: Group therapy, individual therapy, or both? Int J Group Psychother 32:267–282, 1982

Rutan JS, Stone WN: Psychodynamic Group Psychotherapy. Lexington, MA, Collamore Press, 1984

Rutan JS, Alonso A, Groves JE: Understanding defenses in group psychotherapy. Int J Group Psychother 38:459–472, 1988

Ryle A: The focus in brief interpretive psychotherapy: dilemmas, traps and snags as target problems. Br J Psychiatry 134:46–54, 1979

Sachs JS: Negative factors in brief psychotherapy: an empirical assessment. J Consult Clin Psychol 51:557–564, 1983

Salvendy JT: Group psychotherapy training: a quest for standards. Can J Psychiatry 25:394–402, 1980

Saravay SM: A psychoanalytic theory of group development. Int J Group Psychother 28:481–507, 1978

Scheidlinger S: Psychoanalytic Group Dynamics: Basic Readings. New York, International Universities Press, 1980

Scheidlinger S: Presidential Address: On scapegoating in group psychotherapy. Int J Group Psychother 32:131–143, 1982

Scheidlinger S: Focus on Group Psychotherapy. New York, Basic Books, 1983

Scheidlinger S: On interpretation in group psychotherapy: the need for refinement. Int J Group Psychother 37:339–352, 1987

Schutz W: FIRO-B: The Interpersonal Underworld. Palo Alto, CA, Science and Behavioral Books, 1966

Shapiro D: Neurotic Styles. New York, Basic Books, 1965

Shapiro DA, Shapiro D: Meta-analysis of comparative therapy outcome studies: a replication and refinement. Psychol Bull 92:581–604, 1982

Sifneos PE: Short-term Dynamic Psychotherapy, 2nd Edition. New York, Plenum, 1987

Slater PE: Role differentiation in small groups. American Sociological Review 20:300–310, 1955

Slavson SR: Dynamics of Group Psychotherapy. Edited by Schiffer M. New York, Aronson, 1979

Smith ML, Glass GV, Miller TI: The Benefits of Psychotherapy. Baltimore, MD, Johns Hopkins University Press, 1980

Smuts B, Cheney D, Seyfarth R, et al (eds): Primate Societies. Chicago, IL, University of Chicago Press, 1987

Steinbrueck SM, Maxwell SE, Howard GS: A meta-analysis of psychotherapy and drug therapy in the treatment of unipolar depression with adults. J Consult Clin Psychol 51:856–863, 1983

Stone WN, Gustafson JP: Technique in group psychotherapy of narcissistic and borderline patients. Int J Group Psychother 32:29–47, 1982

Stone WN, Whitman RM: Contributions of the psychology of the self to group process and group therapy. Int J Group Psychother 27:343–359, 1977

Strupp HH, Binder JL: Psychotherapy in a New Key: A Guide to Time-Limited Dynamic Psychotherapy. New York, Basic Books, 1984

Strupp HH, Lane TW: An investigation of process and outcome relationships utilizing the Vanderbilt Psychotherapy Process Scale. Paper presented at the meeting of the Society for Psychotherapy Research, Santa Fe, NM, 1988

Strupp HH, Hadley SW, Gomez-Schwartz B: Psychotherapy for Better or Worse: The Problem of Negative Effects. New York, Aronson, 1977

Sullivan HS: The Interpersonal Theory of Psychiatry. New York, Norton, 1953

Toseland RW, Siporin M: When to recommend group treatment: a review of the clinical and group literature. Int J Group Psychother 36:171–201, 1986

Truax CB, Wargo DG, Frank JD, et al: The therapist's contribution to accurate empathy, nonpossessive warmth, and genuineness in psychotherapy. J Clin Psychol 22:331–334, 1966

Tuckman BW: Developmental sequence in small groups. Psychol Bull 63:384–399, 1965

Tyrer P: What's wrong with DSM-III personality disorders? Journal of Personality Disorders 2:281–291, 1988

Waskow IE, Parloff MB: Psychotherapy change measures (DHEW Publ No 74-120). Washington, DC, U.S. Government Printing Office, 1975 (Stock No 1724-00397)

Waxer PH: Short-term group psychotherapy: some principles and techniques. Int J Group Psychother 27:33–42, 1977

Weissman MM, Jarrett RB, Rush JA: Psychotherapy and its relevance to the pharmacotherapy of major depression: a decade later (1976-1985), in Psychopharmacology: The Third Generation of Progress. Edited by Meltzer HY. New York, Raven, 1987

West M, Livesley WJ: Therapist transparency and the frame for group psychotherapy. Int J Group Psychother 36:5–19, 1986

Whitaker DS: Using Groups to Help People. London, Routledge & Kegan Paul, 1985

Whitaker DS, Lieberman MA: Psychotherapy Through the Group Process. New York, Atherton, 1964

Widiger TA, Frances A, Spitzer RL, et al: The DSM-III-R personality disorders: an overview. Am J Psychiatry 145:786–795, 1988

Winston A: The effects of confrontation versus clarification on patient affective and defensive responding. Paper presented at the meeting of the Society for Psychotherapy Research, Santa Fe, NM, 1988

Winston A, Pinsker H, McCullough L: A review of supportive psychotherapy. Hosp Community Psychiatry 37:1105-1114, 1986

Wolf A, Schwartz EK: Psychoanalysis in Groups. New York, Grune and Stratton, 1962

Woods M, Melnick J: A review of group therapy selection criteria. Small Group Behavior 10:155–175, 1979

Wright F, Hoffman XH, Gore EM: Perspectives on scapegoating in primary groups. Group 12:33–44, 1988

Yalom ID: Inpatient Group Psychotherapy. New York, Basic Books, 1983

Yalom ID: The Theory and Practice of Group Psychotherapy, 3rd Edition. New York, Basic Books, 1985

Yalom ID (section ed): Section VI: Group psychotherapy, in Psychiatry Update: American Psychiatric Association Annual Review, Vol 5. Edited by Frances AJ, Hales RE. Washington, DC, American Psychiatric Press, 1986

Index